THE
Middleboro CASEBOOK

THE
Middleboro CASEBOOK

HEALTHCARE STRATEGY
and OPERATIONS

Lee F. Seidel *and* **James B. Lewis**

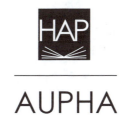

AUPHA

Health Administration Press, Chicago, Illinois
Association of University Programs in Health Administration, Arlington, Virginia

Your board, staff, or clients may also benefit from this book's insight. For more information on quantity discounts, contact the Health Administration Press Marketing Manager at (312) 424-9470.

18   17   16   15   14   5   4   3   2   1

Library of Congress Cataloging-in-Publication Data

Seidel, Lee F.

  The Middleboro casebook : healthcare strategy and operations / Lee F. Seidel and James B. Lewis.
    pages cm
  ISBN 978-1-56793-628-5 (alk. paper)
  1. Integrated delivery of health care--Florida--Hillsboro County. 2. Medical centers--New Hampshire--Hillsboro County. 3. Health services administration--Case studies. I. Lewis, James B. (James Bradley), 1950-
II. Title.
  RA971.S368 2014
  362.109742'8--dc23
                                    2013036545

The paper used in this publication meets the minimum requirements of American National Standard for Information Sciences—Permanence of Paper for Printed Library Materials, ANSI Z39.48-1984. ∞™

Acquisitions editor: Janet Davis; Project manager: Amy Carlton; Cover designer: Christy Collins; Layout: Cepheus Edmondson

Found an error or typo? We want to know! Please e-mail it to hapbooks@ache.org, and put "Book Error" in the subject line.

For photocopying and copyright information, please contact Copyright Clearance Center at www.copyright.com or (978) 750-8400.

Health Administration Press
A division of the Foundation
  of the American College of
  Healthcare Executives
One North Franklin Street
Suite 1700
Chicago, IL 60606-3529
(312) 424-2800

Association of University Programs
  in Health Administration
2000 North 14th Street
Suite 780
Arlington, VA 22201
(703) 894-0940

Dedicated to Mary Fox Arnold (1920–2005), a dynamic professor and healthcare professional. She inspired the early works that eventually led to these cases.

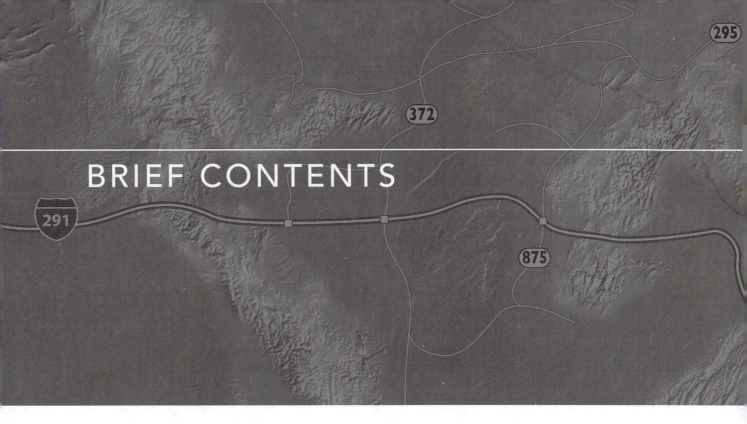

BRIEF CONTENTS

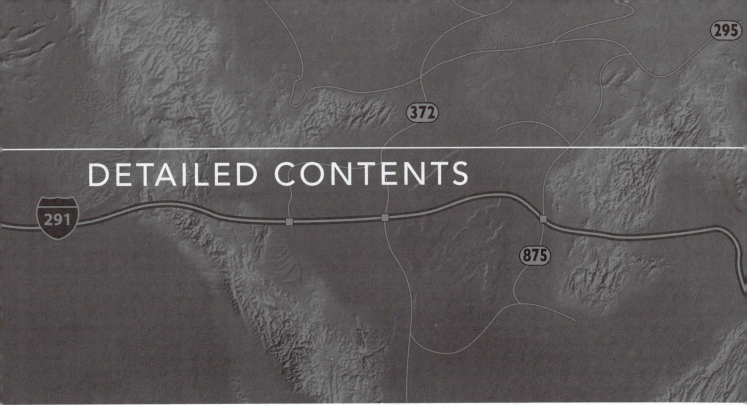

DETAILED CONTENTS

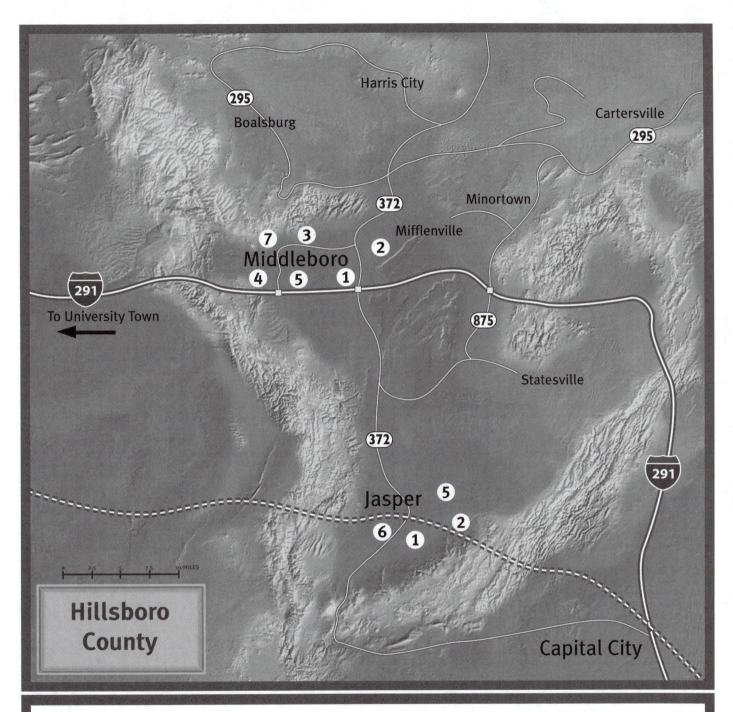

Harris City

295

Boalsburg

Cartersville

295

372

Minortown

7 3

Mifflenville

2

Middleboro

4 5 1

291

To University Town

875

Statesville

372

5

Jasper

2

6 1

291

10 MILES

Capital City

Hillsboro County

Map Legend

Mountains

County and State Roads

Interstate Highway

Interstate Highway (Proposed)

❶ Hillsboro County Home Health Agency (HCHHA)–Middleboro and Jasper

❷ Physician Care Services (PCS)–Mifflenville and Jasper

❸ Middleboro Community Hospital (MCH)–Middleboro

❹ Webster Health System (WHS)–Middleboro

❺ Medical Associates (MA)–Middleboro and Jasper

❻ Jasper Gardens (JG)–Jasper

❼ Hillsboro County Health Department (HCHD)–Middleboro

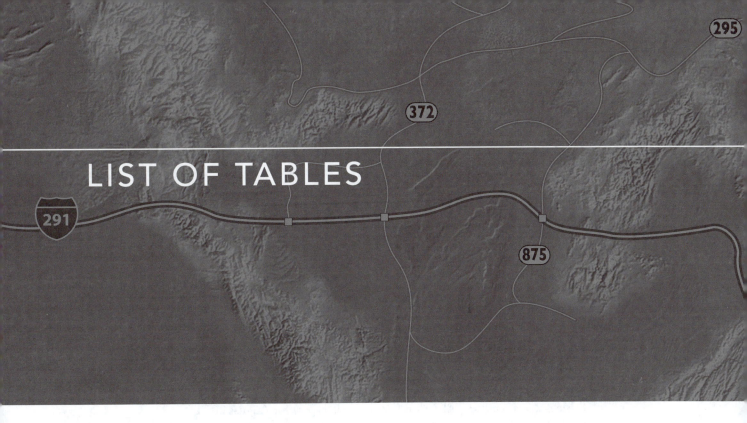

LIST OF TABLES

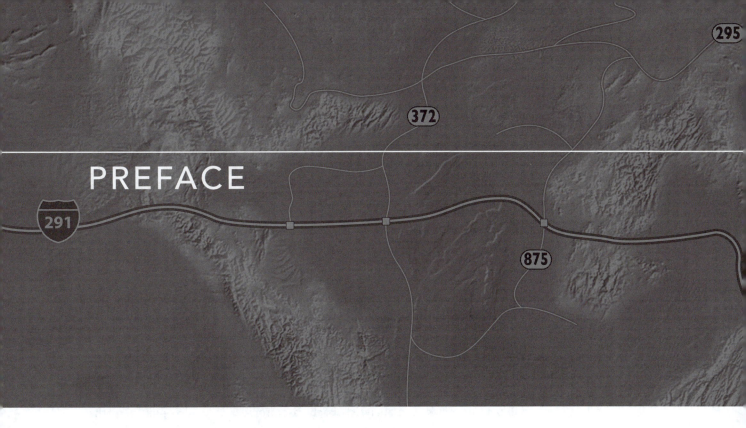

PREFACE

The Middleboro Casebook: Healthcare Strategy and Operations is a flexible and integrated case study focusing on strategy and operations of seven healthcare organizations (two hospitals, a long-term care facility, a home health agency, two physician group practices, and a local health department) located in and around the community of Middleboro. Students are introduced to the community and its demographic, socioeconomic, political, epidemiological, and environmental characteristics. The wealth of data enables students to analyze the community in detail, focusing on those factors that drive the need for and use of healthcare services as well as framing the strategic decisions made by healthcare organizations. Next, students are presented with information about a specific healthcare entity, including its history, governance, organizational structure, programs and services, finances, and particular issues and challenges.

CONCEPT OF THE BOOK

This casebook was developed to bring authentic management and policy issues into the classroom and help students and faculty integrate an academic curriculum in health administration. It provides the basis for identifying many types of problems and issues and formulating management plans and strategies. Since its creation, this book has helped faculty provide a robust integrating seminar as a bridge between academic study and professional practice, and it has provided fuel and substance to courses that address strategic planning and strategic management.

This casebook is unique. It is designed specifically for students of health administration. Each healthcare organization is described in detail in its common community context. Each case requires knowledge from many fields and disciplines. The cases blend the national forces and issues influencing the management of healthcare organizations today with the local forces and issues that make health services management unique. Sensitivity to local events, circumstances, and issues is essential. In *The Middleboro Casebook*—just as in professional practice—excluding the local dimension from the management of health services is impossible. We wanted students, for example, to develop an appreciation and understanding of a community's health needs as part of the process of developing management plans and strategies for the community's healthcare service providers. As such this book presents rich opportunities to embrace a population health approach to strategy.

This book is also a unique academic text. It provides freedom and flexibility to both faculty and students, who can use it to achieve many different types of learning outcomes. For example, students can be asked to define a comprehensive strategy for a specific business unit, or to complete a more focused analysis on a specific aspect of an organization (e.g., financial analysis, marketing analysis). Each case provides a detailed picture of the structure and operation of a different type of healthcare organization. Notice that we have not included specific student assignments. How this book is used is defined by the instructor, who provides the detailed assignment and, if needed, additional information. The instructor's manual includes field-tested assignments for many types of graduate and baccalaureate-level courses and select companion texts. For example, we use one- or two-page "assignment letters" to our students that provide detailed questions and often include additional information. The assignment letters we use with our baccalaureate students are different from the ones we use with our graduate students.

We hope *The Middleboro Casebook* will help students assess and develop their professional repertoire via practice and application.

INTENDED MARKET AND USE

Although this case is new to the national market, it has a history. We have used earlier versions to support instruction at the University of New Hampshire and the business school at the University of Colorado, Denver. It has been used by other faculty in all types of health administration academic programs, including allied and community health, business administration, public health, and community medicine.

The book is an excellent foundation for a capstone course in a baccalaureate or graduate health administration, health policy, or public health curriculum, requiring students to draw from material presented in other courses to refine and apply their strategic thinking. On its own, it can be used as the text for an integrating course or a course in strategic planning or management. Students may find the practical application of their skills more effective for learning than simply reading about the issues.

Also notable is the model developed by Dr. Gary Filerman and the faculty at Georgetown University. They use the cases in multiple foundation courses (e.g., finance, marketing, quality, epidemiology) and then build on this foundation in which students develop strategic and business plans for a specific organization in the case. This model approach, which we call "Middleboro Across the Curriculum," provides depth, breadth, and integration between and among many courses. It has many benefits. Professors Patricia Cloonan, Bernard Horak, and Mary Jane Mastorovich presented a poster on this model at a recent annual meeting of the Association of University Programs in Health Administration (AUPHA), and they deserve recognition for the continued use and evolution of this model.

Helping students integrate their learning is an essential component of an academic curriculum. This casebook provides an alternative to other approaches, including directed field-based consulting, which by its very nature is limited by the constraints of a particular consulting project and may not be truly integrative.

The Middleboro Casebook reflects contemporary plausible reality—a reality influenced by many events and forces. Since the passage of Public Law 111-148, the Patient Protection and Affordable Care Act, health service providers everywhere—including in Middleboro—face new and evolving requirements and issues. The casebook captures this reality, and the assignment process described in the instructor's manual provides a basis to ensure that students are dealing with real current issues.

ANCILLARY MATERIAL

The following materials are available to facilitate the use of this book.

◆ Excel versions of many tables.

◆ An instructor's manual that includes the following resources:

   Section I   Using Middleboro. Presents many issues and suggestions related to problem-based learning and case method teaching applied to this case. This section includes assignment letters, case assignments to create the "problems" for student attention. Using the case across a curriculum is also discussed. This section also includes the authors' perspectives on using the Middleboro cases in a recent baccalaureate membership review with the AUPHA and in a recent accreditation review by the Commission on Accreditation of Healthcare Management Education.

   Section II   Teaching Notes. Provides short essays that describe what the instructor needs to know to use these cases effectively.

Section III   **Suggested Assignments.** Provides recommended assignments in three categories: (1) assignments for each individual case (e.g., Webster Hospital), (2) assignments by subject (e.g., marketing), and (3) assignments designed for specific companion texts:

Dunn, R.T. 2010. *Dunn & Haimann's Healthcare Management*, 9th ed. Chicago: Health Administration Press.

Gapenski, L. C. 2013. *Fundamentals of Healthcare Finance.* Chicago: Health Administration Press.

———. 2012. *Healthcare Finance*, 5th ed. Chicago: Health Administration Press.

Olden, P. C. 2011. *Management of Healthcare Organizations: An Introduction.* Chicago: Health Administration Press.

Thomas, R. K. 2010. *Marketing Health Services.* Chicago: Health Administration Press.

Walston, S. L. 2014. *Strategic Healthcare Management: Planning and Execution.* Chicago: Health Administration Press.

White, K. R., and J. R. Griffith. 2010. *The Well-Managed Healthcare Organization*, 7th ed. Chicago: Health Administration Press.

Zuckerman, A. M. 2012. *Healthcare Strategic Management*, 3rd ed. Chicago: Health Administration Press.

Section IV   **Other Materials.** Includes references and suggested URLs for instructors and students, including references related to oral presentations and business plans.

ACKNOWLEDGMENTS

In addition to those instructors already mentioned, professors Michael Stoto and Robert Friedland at Georgetown University have given much-appreciated advice. To ensure that all cases are realistic, one or more senior healthcare executives have reviewed each case. Trisha, Dennis, Steve, Fritz, Dan, Mike, Tim, and many others have read and reviewed cases from their perspectives as successful managers in the different sectors of our field. Many others have volunteered advice as we have striven to provide our students with an effective foundation. Over the years, the cases have also benefited from the many comments and suggestions provided by other faculty, senior healthcare executives, and students, especially the students in the executive MBA program at the University of Colorado, Denver. Professor Errol Biggs, director of the executive MBA in health administration at CU Denver, deserves special recognition and our appreciation.

Our interest in this type of casebook traces its roots to the classic study, *Middletown: A Study of American Culture,* by Helen and Robert Lynd (1929). We hope that the Lynds forgive us for using a play on the name of their comprehensive community study.

We alone are responsible for any errors, including any errors in the many tables of data.

CONCLUSION

Middleboro, Hillsboro County, and all the organizations and people described in the cases are fictitious. Any similarity to real people and places is merely an unintended consequence. Also, the casebook has no preconceived outcomes. Management is both art and science. We hope readers use both to define and address problems and issues and plan to enhance access, quality, and lower costs.

As you enter each case, remember to peel it like an onion. Read it over and look for connections. Explore it. Think about it. Cases must be read numerous times. Use your managerial repertoire to sort through the facts and issues. You must decide what is important and what is trivial. Trust and test your instincts as a manager. Use the case to integrate, broaden, and sharpen your analytical and intuitive abilities as a professional manager of health services. Connect the dots you think are important. Read the entire case before you begin working on any single facet of the case. Information relevant to one organization is frequently included in the case of another organization.

One cannot be an accomplished musician merely by studying music theory. You need to apply and test your repertoire of skills and insights. *The Middleboro Casebook* can help as you mature beyond the silos of learning that characterize higher education. Integrating your managerial repertoire across these silos and applying it to realistic issues is a challenging test. Few get it "right" the first time. Remember that truly integrating your learning is your responsibility; faculty can only provide the opportunity, support, and general direction. Most students—regardless of their backgrounds—both love and hate this casebook. For some, it has too much information. For others, not enough. Over many years, however, most students agree that using it has validated, changed, and sharpened their professional skills, values, and insights as they strive to be proficient managers of organized health services. Health services management requires preparation involving both education and experience. We hope this case provides some of each. Just for the record, Middleboro, Jasper, and Hillsboro County are not in New Hampshire.

Welcome to Middleboro and Hillsboro County. It is midnight on December 31, 2014, and 2015 has begun.

Lee F. Seidel, PhD
James B. Lewis, ScD

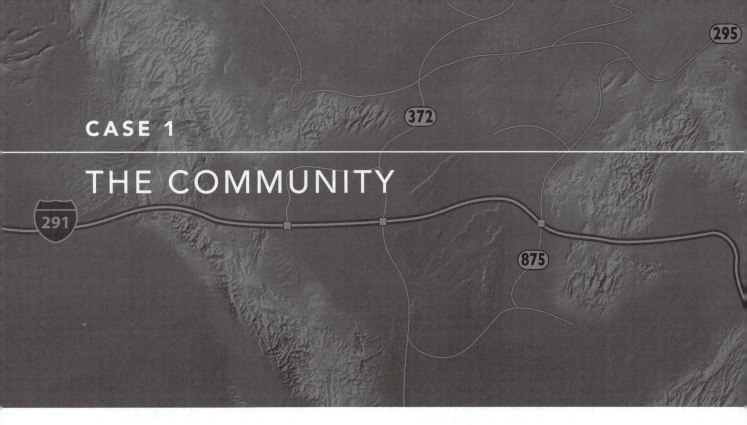

CASE 1
THE COMMUNITY

Many people regard Hillsboro County as a comfortable place to raise a family. The area is known for its social and economic stability. While the residents are generally aware of national and world events, local news about the activities of youth teams, social fraternal organizations, church outings, and high school sports dominates the local media. Multiple generations of families live in Middleboro and the surrounding towns comprising Hillsboro County.

DEMOGRAPHIC CHARACTERISTICS

Middleboro and Hillsboro County are classified as nonmetropolitan areas. Middleboro has been the economic, political and social hub for Hillsboro County. The average family size is 2.77 people. Basic demographic data are given in Table 1.1 Hillsboro County Population, Table 1.2 Hillsboro County Population by Race, and Table 1.3 Age Profile for Hillsboro County by Sex.

The other major community in this area is the city of Jasper, located 23 miles to the southeast of Middleboro. Jasper is a growing community that has experienced the benefit of being close to Capital City, the state capital. Jasper is slowly becoming a commuter town for Capital City and is continuing to develop as an economy that is independent from Middleboro. The population of Jasper recently surpassed that of Middleboro.

GEOGRAPHIC CHARACTERISTICS

Surrounded on two sides by mountains, access to Middleboro is limited to rail service (freight), bus, and highway. The majority of private and commercial travel is by automobile, bus, and truck. Served by an auxiliary four-lane, east–west interstate highway, Middleboro is 45 miles northwest of Capital City and 70 miles east of the location of the state university (University Town). The commercial airport is located in Capital City. The interstate highway is typically closed an average of three days per year because of weather conditions. The mountains on the east and west of Middleboro make winter travel outside the area especially difficult. North and south of Middleboro are fertile valleys known for their agricultural activities.

Outside of the towns of Middleboro and Jasper, the population lives in small, scattered villages. From these communities, rural county and state highways are the only transportation links to Middleboro. The area has limited bus service. Middleboro serves as the regional transportation hub; the bus station in Middleboro has connections to major population centers in the state. Jasper is also served by this bus system. Recently, a commuter bus system began linking Jasper with Capital City.

The county stretches 45 miles to the north, 15 miles to the west, 18 miles to the east, and 37 miles to the south of Middleboro. Table 1.4 indicates the miles between communities located in the county. In the total area, 71 percent of the land is developed; the remainder is forest, state park land, and rivers. This area experiences four distinct seasons. Tourists find it especially attractive during the fall and spring. Sports of all types play an important role in the life of the community.

The City of Middleboro is located on Swift River, which was instrumental in the commercial development of the city in the early 1800s. Before 1900, the Swift River and the commercial barges that traversed it were the community's primary link with the rest of the state. Now the river is used for recreational purposes, and some limited redevelopment of the riverside property has begun.

The river divides Middleboro into two almost equal parts. The north side of the river is the site of the central business district, large manufacturing plants, the railroad station, older residential neighborhoods, and the county government. During the 1970s, federal funds were used to develop low-income housing on the north side. On the south side, which is closer to the interstate highway, the residential neighborhoods are generally newer. The south side contains the new high school and small shopping centers. To date, the City of Middleboro has not approved any development—residential or commercial—in the vacant 150-acre area adjacent to the interstate highway.

SOCIAL AND EDUCATIONAL CHARACTERISTICS

The population of the area is predominately of German, Irish, and English extraction. Racial minority groups comprise about 9 percent of the population. Most of the

African-Americans arrived in the 1960s, and most of the other racial groups arrived in the late 1970s. About 10.6 percent of households are headed by a female.

The median education level of the population over 25 years of age is 10.7 years. Approximately 21 percent of the population has completed college, and 53 percent has completed high school. The current dropout rate from area high schools is 9 percent, an improvement over the 17 percent rate experienced 10 years ago.

Middleboro is the site of numerous elementary schools (grades K–6), a regional middle school (grades 7–8), and a high school (grades 9–12) that serve students from Middleboro. Other communities can send their children to these schools using tuition arrangements on a space-available basis. Although all the schools are owned and operated by the City of Middleboro, a separately elected Middleboro School Board makes educational policy. One-third of the nine-member school board is elected each year in a special school district election. Each year, the Middleboro School Board submits a recommended budget for consideration by the Middleboro City Council. The city council approves the school budget before it is submitted, as part of the city's total budget, for voter approval. All employees of the Middleboro School Department, except the superintendent of schools, Dr. Sam Drucker, are unionized. Janet Simon is currently the chairperson of the school board, a position she has held for the past ten years. The new $18.5 million high school in Middleboro opened last year after being considered by the city council for about eight years.

Jasper is the site of numerous elementary schools, a regional middle school (grades 5–8), and a small high school (grades 9–12). A state-supported junior college will open in 2016. A five-member elected school board that is independent of the city governs the Jasper Regional Educational Cooperative. Each year, this school board submits a recommended budget directly to the voters. Once approved, the City of Jasper is obligated to collect the approved funds using local taxes. The Jasper Regional Education Cooperative has expressed interest in working with the state to develop a regional vocational high school to complement the new Hillsboro County Junior College.

State University (SU) in University Town has a nursing, public health, and allied health school connected to its relatively large liberal arts and agricultural schools. SU is the land-grant university within the state. It has 19,000 students, making it the largest public university in the state. A private liberal arts college of 1,000 students is located in Capital City. SU also maintains a small branch campus in Capital City.

Church membership remains strong in the area. Aside from their religious influence, churches sponsor many of the youth sports leagues and are the site of many social gatherings.

Local chapters of Rotary International meet monthly in Middleboro and Jasper. The AARP also maintains a chapter in Middleboro. The local chapter of American Red Cross, located in Middleboro, sponsors monthly blood drives throughout the area

Once statistics are adjusted for demographic characteristics, crime rates are 10 percent below national averages for nonmetropolitan areas.

POLITICAL CHARACTERISTICS

Middleboro and the surrounding area are politically conservative. Unlike other areas in the state, the same political party has dominated this area for the past 45 years. Its politicians have gained statewide political power by consistently being reelected to office. Middleboro is especially proud that the area's representative to the United States Congress, James Giles, is a Middleboro native who retains his law practice in town.

Middleboro is governed by a six-member city council that is elected every two years; by tradition, the member receiving the largest number of popular votes is appointed by the council to serve as mayor. Although the office's powers are mostly ceremonial, the mayor has the ability to influence decisions by presiding over council meetings and by making appointments to boards and commissions. Keith Edwards, a local retailer, has held the position of mayor for 17 years. Other members of the Middleboro City Council are Frederick Washburn, Diana Story, David Alley, Patricia Hood, and Michael York. The largest department of the city is the school department, and the second largest is public works. Michael York is the council member with lead responsibilities on all issues and programs involving healthcare.

The City of Middleboro has recently begun legal action to block the licensing of three group homes in Middleboro for the developmentally disabled population. Group Homes, Inc., a national corporation, would be the owner and operator of these homes, based on a contract with the state. According to Mayor Edwards, the Hillsboro County Health Department has failed to consider the serious implications of building these homes in Middleboro. Mayor Edwards advocates that the application for licensure be turned down on grounds related to negative community impact.

Middleboro is also the county seat for Hillsboro County. Three county commissioners elected by the population at large govern Hillsboro County. While the county level of government is not a powerful political subdivision in this region of the country, it does control the court system, the penal system, and the registry of motor vehicles, and it provides some human service programs. Hillsboro County owns and operates a nursing home located in Middleboro. It is a major county employer in the area. The current commissioners are Janet Ruseski, Bill Nelligan, and Bill Harrison.

A 12-member town council and a mayor govern Jasper. Both are elected for four-year terms. William Hines is mayor, a position he has held for the past nine years. The town council employs a professional city manager (Susan Giles-Harrison). The Jasper Industrial Development Authority (JIDA), authorized by the voters approximately 15 years ago, is a subunit of the town council and has the authority to issue long-term bonds to support industrial development in Jasper. Susan Giles-Harrison also serves as executive director of JIDA. Approximately two years ago, JIDA formed a special committee to consider the feasibility of a hospital located on JIDA property that was owned and operated by the town. This committee is chaired by Sharon Lee, the spouse of a Jasper physician, a member of the town council, and a former consultant for a national consulting firm that specialized in healthcare. Other members of this committee include Mayor Hines and town councilor Ed Hicks. Giles-Harrison provides staff support for this committee.

Under a program supported by the federal Department of Homeland Security, the mayors of all the communities in Hillsboro County and their fire and police officials have created a special task force to estimate "surge capacity." Officials from both hospitals have also attended these meetings. The task force continues to update its estimate of potential locations and beds that could be used in an emergency and mass casualty situation. The governor's office has also supported this project with funding for a countywide assessment of surge capacity by State University.

Initial findings and results indicate the following:

◆ Hillsboro County has at least 385 hotel and motel rooms available.

◆ Public schools should be able to hold approximately 4,500 citizens, although none has provisions for emergencies.

◆ The disaster plans for both hospitals have not been coordinated. Each has its own plan and has estimated that it can accommodate at least 150 to 180 percent of its inpatient capacity for one week.

◆ No area-wide centralized communication system or command and control system is able to direct resources and responses in the face of a significant disaster.

The more comprehensive assessment and plan is expected in six months.

Since 2009 Hillsboro County has sponsored a Community Emergency Response Team (CERT) Program to educate people about disaster preparedness for hazards that may arise in the area, such as fires, floods, and weather-related disasters. Classes are held three times a year, and to date approximately 120 local residents have completed training. Program instructors have been drawn from local police and fire departments, both local hospitals, and the health department.

For the past five years the state legislature has considered making the state a "right to work state" that would limit the power of labor unions. Although the law was not passed, last year the law did secure 52 percent approval in the state senate. The current governor has indicated that if the legislation passes the state legislature he would veto it. His political opponents have stated that they support right-to-work legislation.

ECONOMIC CHARACTERISTICS

The tax profile of the area reflects the conservative nature of the community. Increases in property taxes have just barely kept pace with inflation. The state has both a graduated income tax and a sales tax. By state law any incorporated city is allowed to add a 0.5

percent local sales tax to the state sales tax. The Middleboro City Council has repeatedly rejected all proposals to do this.

Middleboro is the site of important wholesale and retail trade in the county. Major companies include manufacturing, finance, and service industries. Jasper is also establishing itself as a manufacturing center. Agriculture, which once dominated the area, now accounts for 20 percent of the area's income and 16 percent of all employment. Manufacturing accounts for 32 percent of income and 30 percent of employment. Per capita income is 9 percent below the national average. Fourteen percent of Hillsboro County's population falls below the federal poverty level. Note that in Capital City this figure is 18 percent.

Local banks estimate that approximately 8 percent of the single homes in the county have outstanding mortgages greater than their current market value. The regional foreclosure rate is 1 percent greater than the national rate.

Three of Middleboro's manufacturing companies employ nearly 20 percent of the workforce, down approximately 7 percent from five years ago. Carlstead Rayon is a privately controlled textile corporation and employs 6.1 percent of the workforce. River Industries, a division of National Auto Technology, manufactures rubber products for automobiles. Over a three-year period, it has reduced its workforce by 7 percent. The third major manufacturing company is Master Tractor, formerly a division of United Agricultural Supply. Master Tractor was recently sold to a Japanese firm that has indicated that some component parts for tractors will be imported from offshore and South American suppliers. Master Tractor is a leader in the market for small tractors. It employs 4.6 percent of the workforce. All three companies are unionized and provide employees a choice of health insurance plans. Within the past year, executives from the three industries have been meeting informally to discuss the growing problem of increasing healthcare costs. At the most recent meeting, the companies agreed that a more formal structure would be established to study the problems and to devise possible approaches to reverse the trend. They also agreed that the unions representing employees of all three employers would be invited to participate in the talks.

Carlstead Rayon, River Industries, and Master Tractor are all located adjacent to rail service.

Blue Bear Ale, a popular statewide microbrewery owned by a national corporation, is currently examining sites in Middleboro and Mifflenville to establish a new regional brewery. Three years ago, US Parts, a division of a national corporation, which manufactures components for large air conditioning units, relocated to Jasper. Today this company employs 3.2 percent of the area's workforce.

Table 1.5 and Table 1.6 summarize healthcare benefits provided to employees by major area corporations. Table 1.7 estimates insurance coverage throughout the county.

Last year, National Yearbook, a corporation headquartered in a major western city, established a modern printing and manufacturing plant in Jasper using resources provided by JIDA. This company specializes in manufacturing yearbooks for colleges and high schools. Although its current workforce is small, with only 81 employees, National

Yearbook has indicated that employment should increase 10 percent for each of the next ten years as it reduces its existing regional manufacturing sites and concentrates its entire North American manufacturing at the Jasper plant. National Yearbooks is not unionized and offers a full range of health insurance options to its full-time employees.

The Jasper Industrial Park, located on the western boundary of Jasper, is also the site for the regional warehouse of Office Pro—a retail and wholesale provider of office supplies and office furniture.

Agriculture and construction companies in this area are primarily small businesses. Chicken Farms, Inc., located in Harris City, is a national corporation specializing in raising chickens for fast food restaurants. It recently began to acquire family farms in the area and has announced plans to locate a processing plant somewhere in Hillsboro County.

Housing construction permits have steadily declined over the last seven years. The housing stock is considered old, except in Jasper, by both national and state standards.

The area has one state chartered commercial bank, the Middleboro Trust Company, that has offices in Middleboro, Mifflenville, Statesville, Harris City, and Jasper. The area also has four small savings and loans institutions, which were started principally to provide capital to the agricultural sector. To avoid insolvency 12 years ago, the Merchants Bank of Capital City acquired the Carterville Bank (savings and loan). Harry Carter, the bank's president, was a prominent politician at that time and was subsequently convicted of investor fraud.

Major capital financing is available through the Middleboro Trust Company, a correspondent bank of a major national financial institution, or through a commercial bank located in Capital City. Bankers' Cooperative, a multistate commercial bank headquartered in another state, has recently announced plans to expand into Jasper.

Within the past two months the Hillsboro County Chamber of Commerce sponsored a full-day meeting on the potential implications associated with the Patient Protection and Affordable Care Act (ACA). Following this meeting Carlstead Rayon and three other major employers indicated that they would consider limiting or eliminating employee health insurance as a benefit and pay the federal penalties as established by this law. Carlstead Rayon also indicated that its parent company is considering shifting all health and medical insurances to a Taft Hartley Health Fund. Under this approach, the union controls all health and welfare benefits. Union members and employers pay the expenses associated with the provision of services. The fund specifies coverage and administers all claims and payments.

The chamber will continue to hold these meetings so that employers understand the implications associated with federal and state policy changes.

MEDIA

The major newspaper in the area is the *Middleboro Sentinel*. It has a daily as well as a Sunday edition and maintains a comprehensive website. The newspaper's circulation is approximately 22,000 for the daily and 8,200 for the Sunday edition. Three years ago

National News Stands, Inc., a national owner and operator of local newspapers, acquired it. Jack Donnelly remains the editor of the paper, a position he has held for 16 years. In Jasper, the *Capital City News* reaches approximately 25 percent of all households. Their rates are similar to the *Middleboro Sentinel*'s.

Three local radio stations in Middleboro, AM-75, AM-1220 and FM-89.7, also provide coverage of news events. TV Channel 32 is an independent station located in Middleboro. It provides network as well as independent programs. Affiliates of national television networks are located in Capital City; most residents can receive them through the airways. Cable TV is available in Middleboro, Mifflenville, and Jasper and includes the normal range of broadcasting stations as well as local public service programs.

MEDICAL RESOURCES

HILLSBORO COUNTY HEALTH DEPARTMENT

The county health department is located in Middleboro and provides services throughout the county. Dr. Tim Taylor is the current chairperson of the County Board of Health. This 12-person board is appointed for overlapping five-year terms by the Hillsboro County Commissioners. John Snow, MPH, directs and manages the health department. Other professional employees include registered nurses, public health assistants, and individuals with special expertise in public health. The department's responsibilities focus on the distribution of state funds to local health agencies, immunizations, environmental health, the oversight of Manorhaven (a long-term care facility), and the implementation of county health priorities using county tax revenues. The Hillsboro County Health Department, in cooperation with a statewide data system, also gathers vital and mortality statistics which, in turn, are sent to the state. The department provides the data as part of its annual report to the county commissioners.

Table 1.8 provides the estimated number of active cases of sexually transmitted disease and types of cancer. Table 1.9 provides statistics related to AIDS and HIV. Table 1.10 includes data on diabetes. Table 1.11 compares county BRFSS (Behavioral Risk Factor Surveillance System) data with state and regional data. Table 1.12 reports the prevalence of asthma. Table 1.13 reports the Healthy People 2020 goals and 2010 state accomplishments.

HILLSBORO COUNTY HOME HEALTH AGENCY, INC.

This home health agency was formerly known as the Middleboro Home Health Agency. It is a tax-exempt, Medicare-certified organization that provides home-based services throughout the county. The agency, with offices in Middleboro and Jasper, also sponsors community health and health-promotion activities with funds provided by the towns and cities in the area, Hillsboro County, and United Appeal. Maternal and child health programs are funded by a grant from the state's department of Health and Human Services. Martha Washington, RN, is the director. Janet Myer is president of the board of directors.

Medical Associates

Medical Associates is a multispecialty medical group of physicians. Founded in 1961, it has offices in downtown Middleboro and in Jasper. It is a for-profit, private corporation organized as a professional partnership. All physicians are board certified and maintain active medical staff privileges at area hospitals. Medical Associates provides specialty and subspecialty care on an ambulatory care basis. Recently, the Jasper location established limited ambulatory surgical services. It contracts with Wythe Laboratories in Capital City for medical tests. Walter Graham is the senior administrator.

Middleboro Community Hospital

This hospital is a fully licensed, tax-exempt, acute care hospital on the north side of Middleboro. It was founded in 1890. Most of the current beds are located in a wing constructed in 1962 and 1966 with the assistance of federal Hill-Burton funds. A full range of diagnostic, outpatient, therapeutic, and emergency medical services are provided, including a cancer treatment program. Adjacent to the hospital is the Middleboro Medical Office Building. Ample parking is available for both the hospital and the medical office building. Table 1.14 provides hospital discharges and patient days. James Higgens is the administrator of the hospital. Although it is licensed for 272 beds, the hospital has reduced its inpatient capacity over the last five years to reduce costs and adjust to new hospital utilization patterns.

Physician Care Services, Inc.

Physician Care Services (PCS) owns and operates two urgent care centers, one in Mifflenville and the other in Jasper. The corporation employs physicians and other professionals and provides walk-in ambulatory care and a full range of diagnostic services, including an occupational health program. PCS is a private, for-profit corporation. Dr. Stephen Tobias is president and CEO.

Webster Health System

Webster Health System owns and operates a fully accredited, tax-exempt, osteopathic hospital in Middleboro adjacent to the interstate highway. Named after its founder Dr. Edward W. Webster, this health system was founded as a hospital in 1930. The hospital has an active medical staff of osteopathic physicians and makes use of many other physicians with consulting privileges from Osteopathic Medical Center (OMC) in Capital City. Table 1.14 provides hospital discharges and patient days. Janice Masterman is the administrator of the hospital. Six years ago, Webster Hospital changed its name to Webster Health System and became an affiliate corporation of Osteopathic Hospitals of America, Inc. (OHA). Under this affiliation, OMC and OHA have agreed to supervise the management of the Webster Health System, provide joint purchasing and supply chain opportunities and capital in return for an exclusive contract for all medically appropriate referrals. Since executing the agreement, Webster Hospital has established Quick Med, a walk-in ambulatory care clinic adjacent to its emergency department, recruited physicians, and expanded all services related to birthing. The tax-exempt hospital and a for-profit organization jointly owned by the hospital and members of the medical staff constitute the Webster Health System.

The number and type of physicians in Hillsboro County are described on Table 1.15. Except for the physicians affiliated with Medical Associates, the area has multiple single-specialty and solo medical practices.

AREA LONG-TERM CARE FACILITIES

The Carter Home is located north of Middleboro and Jasper near Mifflenville and is a tax-paying, 150-bed long-term care facility that qualifies for both Medicare and Medicaid. Jack H. Carter has been president of the Carter Home Corporation, Inc., for the past 20 years and is currently the administrator of the Carter Home. Recently, the Carter Home Corporation announced plans to add Carter Village, an assisted living facility with 150 two-bedroom apartments with a congregate meal facility, 24-hour access to nursing services, access to physical and occupational therapists, and van service to shopping areas in Middleboro.

Jasper Gardens, located in Jasper, is a private, tax-paying, 110-bed long-term care facility. It qualifies for Medicare, Medicaid, all insurances, and self-pay. Jefferson Partners LLC of Capital City owns it. Jayne Winters is the licensed administrator. She is a graduate of an eastern university and holds an undergraduate degree in health services management.

Manorhaven is a 110-bed long-term care facility in Middleboro, owned and operated by Hillsboro County. Services qualify for both Medicare and Medicaid reimbursement. Manorhaven operates a limited adult day care program for residents in Middleboro. Jennifer Jones has been the administrator for the past eight years.

Rock Creek is a private 126-bed long-term care facility located north of Mifflenville near Harris City. It qualifies for Medicaid insurance. No Medicare patients are served. Five years ago a statewide proprietary chain purchased it. Its current administrator is John Lipman.

Senior Living of Mifflenville is an assisted-living facility located between Middleboro and Mifflenville. Two types of living arrangements are offered. In the 45-unit assisted living facility, residents rent private one- and two-bedroom units. Each unit has a small kitchen. Senior Living provides congregate meals, transportation services, and a full recreational program. In the adult home, 125 residents are provided either private or semiprivate room accommodation. A 24-hour nursing staff provides supervision. Senior Living of Mifflenville opened four years ago and is owned and operated by a national corporation. The adult home is not a licensed nursing home.

OTHER HEALTH SERVICES

Middleboro Counseling Center, located in Middleboro, was established in 1968 as one of the region's original nonprofit community mental health centers. The director, Dr. Dean Tibbitts, is a psychologist specializing in juvenile emotional disorders. The center employs four full-time counselors. It has contracted with Webster Hospital for emergency psychiatric services. Involuntary psychiatric admissions are sent to the state mental hospital in Capital City. The center provides group and individual counseling and crisis intervention for both adult and juvenile populations.

Gateway Health Services is a professional partnership of state-certified mental health counselors. It has office locations in Mifflenville and Jasper. It provides individual and group therapy. Staff includes psychologists, social workers, family and marriage therapists, and counselors. Services focus on a full range of diseases and issues including anxiety, depression, and addiction.

A 2010 study conducted by State University concluded that Hillsboro County has an "adequate number" of mental health and family counselors. Most of these counselors work as solo practitioners.

The state supports three inpatient psychiatric institutions. The closest to Hillsboro County is 45 miles west of Capital City.

Valley Hospice, Inc., is a tax-exempt hospice that is totally dependent on charitable contributions from the community. It maintains an office in Middleboro and employs Mary Care, RN, as its half-time executive director and a part-time social worker. It recruits and trains volunteers to provide emotional support to adult cancer patients and their families. Jack Donnelly is the president of the board of directors and the Reverend Philip Martin is the vice president. All funds are donated.

Churches in both Middleboro and Jasper coordinate and provide Meals on Wheels. Under this program, homebound elderly receive a delivered hot lunch.

Prehospital services are provided by a variety of providers. In Middleboro, the fire department provides emergency services staffed with emergency medical technicians (EMTs). In Jasper, the fire department uses paramedics to provide emergency services. Other communities rely on volunteer fire departments and volunteer emergency services, some of which require basic EMT certification. This year the county has established a countywide 911 emergency dispatch system.

Statewide Blue Cross and Blue Shield is headquartered in Capital City. Also located in Capital City are state chapters and associations, including the following:

- Alzheimer's Association

- AARP

- American Cancer Society

- American Diabetes Association

- American Heart Association

- American Lung Association

- Brain Injury Association

- Epilepsy Foundation

- Muscular Dystrophy Association

- National Mental Health Association

- United Cerebral Palsy Association

It should be noted that the statewide Alzheimer's Association has publicly expressed its priority to establish a membership in Middleboro and throughout Hillsboro County.

Two medical schools are located in this state. The one supported by the state is on its eastern boundary and the other—a private osteopathic medical school—is on its northern boundary. Both are located in major cities and are more than 250 miles away from Capital City. Over the past 30 years, the hospitals in Capital City have become major referral centers for community hospitals located within a 100- to 125-mile geographic circle. The two largest hospitals in Capital City—Capital City General and OMC—maintain teaching affiliations with the medical schools in the state.

Dentists in private practice throughout the county provide dental services. Most are single independent practitioners. The county has approximately 42.0 dentists per 100,000 people. There are 20.3 veterinarians per 100,000 in the county. Registered nurses number 811.4 and physician assistants 27.0 per 100,000, respectively. Hillsboro County has six licensed mortuaries, four in Middleboro and two in Jasper.

Table 1.16 provides vital statistics. Tables 1.17 and 1.18 provide mortality statistics.

STATE REGULATIONS

The state has maintained a Certificate of Need (CON) law for all acute and specialty hospitals and long-term care facilities that receive Medicaid and/or Medicare. Home health agencies were exempted from the law seven years ago. Also specifically excluded from the law are private physician offices, clinics, and dispensaries for employees and health maintenance organizations. The thresholds for application of CON are $4 million for major medical equipment, $10 million for new construction, any transfer of ownership, and any increase in the number of licensed bed size equal to or greater than 15 beds or 20 percent of the facility (whichever is less). CON proposals are evaluated based on the proposal's ability to better address the needs of the service area, immediate and long-term financial viability, and quality-of-care implications.

CON applications are forwarded to the Commissioner of Health and Welfare of the state and analyzed by the State Bureau of Healthcare Services. The CON board renders the final decision. The governor, based on recommendation of the state legislature, appoints this seven-member board. Jack Carter, the only local representative on this board, owns a nursing home in Hillsboro County. The governor, working with a committee in the state legislature, will be issuing recommendations on whether CON should be reauthorized, changed, or allowed to lapse as a state statute.

RECENT COMMUNITY CONCERNS AND ISSUES

Local political leaders have long recognized that the Middleboro area is economically stagnant. They have discussed the need for a major industrial park adjacent to the interstate highway. Local business leaders, however, have resisted this venture. They have suggested that the public funds designated for this activity need to be invested in improvements in the central business district to bolster the city's existing retail trade business. As a result of these competing views, Middleboro has not invested in developing either.

The entire area has been affected by the national downturn in the traditional industrial and manufacturing sector. The current unemployment rate in the county is 4.4 percentage points higher than the state's overall rate. Most of the county's unemployment is in the Middleboro area.

Almost 15 years ago, a flood hit Middleboro. The flood heavily damaged Carlstead Rayon. While some of this damage has been repaired, the corporation did not return to full production. It elected to use the insurance settlement to open a new production facility in another state with a right-to-work law and to switch some production to an overseas location. In an emergency settlement one month before the corporation was about to completely close its Middleboro facility, it agreed to maintain a scaled down manufacturing operation in Middleboro as long as all real estate taxes were waived in perpetuity and that the state provide it industrial development bonds for capital acquisition. Although this settlement did save a significant number of jobs, local and state political leaders continue to be criticized for the terms of the agreement. Earlier this year, the *Middleboro Sentinel* ran a series of stories on the environmental hazards caused by Carlstead Rayon's questionable handling of waste materials through the years. Finally, about one month ago, the County

Health Department requested a health consultation of the Carlstead site by the Agency for Toxic Substances and Disease Registry of the US Department of Health and Human Services' Public Health Service. The consultation report is anticipated within the next two months, and it is expected to conclude that portions of the Carlstead operation will be designated as a hazardous waste site, subject to remediation requirements.

Carlstead Rayon has recently informed the City of Middleboro that it wants a 25 percent reduction in the price it pays for city water.

The Middleboro Town Council has repeatedly asked all tax-exempt healthcare providers to make a payment in lieu of taxes (PILT) to cover municipal services. Last year, Steven Local ran for city council with this as his only issue, promising the voters to convince the hospitals and other healthcare "free riders" that they must "pay their fair share" or face consequences, including court action. He lost the election by 21 votes and has vowed to return next year with an even stronger campaign. It should be noted that for the past five years Hillsboro County has received an annual payment of approximately $28,000 under the federal PILT program (PL 103-79).

For the past five years, Middleboro politics have been dominated by three issues: the increases in local property taxes, the cost of schools, and the use of local funds included in Medicaid to pay for abortions. Generally issues involving economic development have not characterized local political campaigns.

Over the past three years, major industrial development has occurred in Jasper with the arrival of US Parts, a division of a national corporation, which manufactures components for large air conditioning units. Today this company occupies almost 60 percent of the Jasper Industrial Park established five years ago. National Yearbooks, Inc., is expected to fill the remaining capacity in this industrial park within the next five years. Political officials in Middleboro continue to be criticized for letting Jasper "beat out" Middleboro for these major employers.

In 18 months the state will open a new moderate security prison southwest of Jasper. The prison will have a capacity of 600 inmates and is part of the state's plan to develop regional prison facilities. Seven years ago, Sam Donovan, a state senator from Jasper, began the community effort to secure this prison for the Jasper area. It is expected to become another major employer in the area.

Issues involving growth have dominated politics in Jasper. While the entire community seems satisfied with the success of the industrial development authority, many are equally dissatisfied with the impact this development has had on municipal services and the local education system. Responsible Growth, a group of 100 concerned citizens, was organized two years ago to voice these concerns and last year succeeded in electing two of its members, Jennifer Kip and Alan Simpson, to the city council. Both expressed concern that Jasper was too quickly becoming a commuter town for Capital City.

National Development Corp. has recently presented the Town of Jasper's planning board with a proposal for an 800-unit subdivision of moderately priced housing located on land adjacent to the new interstate road. The proposal holds the developer responsible for all infrastructures.

Four months ago, Representative James Giles announced—with the governor—that a new four-lane interstate highway would be built between Capital City and Jasper. This road will shorten the travel distance to 15 miles. Rep. Giles acknowledged that this project would inject numerous new jobs into the local economy and would provide Jasper the transportation link it has needed for the past 15 years. It should be completed in three years. Some have criticized this road construction project as just a way to get more people to and from athletic events at State University, as the road is designed to eventually link University Town with Capital City. The Jasper City Council, including members Kip and Simpson, recently voted to approve the zoning application for a major shopping mall complex adjacent to this new road and at the edge of Jasper, approximately five miles from downtown Jasper and ten miles from the boundary of Capital City.

When contacted by the mayor of Middleboro, Rep. Giles indicated that this new interstate was unlikely to ever extend to Middleboro. Long-term plans have this road intersecting the existing east–west interstate highway in University Town. Rep. Giles did indicate, however, that he would discuss with the governor whether state funds exist to upgrade the road between Jasper and Middleboro to a limited access highway.

Under recent federal legislation, the state Department of Transportation issued a feasibility study involving a commuter rail link between Jasper and Capital City. The plan indicates that such a system may be feasible if Jasper continues to grow at its current rate over the next five to seven years.

Citizens Against Abortions has also developed as a small but vocal political force in Jasper. On three occasions demonstrators have picketed the offices of area physicians known to have performed abortions at hospitals in either Middleboro or Capital City. TV Action 12, the evening news broadcast of the largest TV station in Capital City, covered two of these demonstrations in Jasper. This group has announced plans to begin picketing area hospitals. The local newspaper has estimated that this organization, however, has no more than 35 members.

Leaders from Harris City, Boalsburg, Minortown, and Carterville have begun to meet monthly to discuss common concerns. They have recently issued a statement directed toward the Hillsboro county commissioners. They indicated that too many county resources were being devoted to help the southern part of the county at the expense of the smaller communities north of the interstate highway.

Community philanthropy has declined in this entire area. As a condition associated with the receipt of funds from United Appeal, a nonprofit agency must forgo any independent fund-raising, although it can accept individual gifts. Over the past ten years, the rate of giving has declined 30 percent, and the amount disbursed by United Appeal has declined by 16 percent. Even though all large industries as well as many small employers cooperate with the United Appeal, all measures suggest that philanthropy has significantly declined.

In the most recent legislative session, a law was passed eliminating the ability of insurers doing business in the state to exclude people from coverage due to preexisting conditions. This action was taken independently from the federal ACA that was passed with similar provisions coming into effect in 2014. In addition, debate is ongoing in the statehouse on a small-group health insurance reform bill. If passed, small employers in the state—defined here as having fewer than ten employees—would have the opportunity to participate in health insurance purchasing pools, designed to provide them with access to coverage at a lower rate than previous arrangements. The state decided not to participate in the insurance exchange stipulated by ACA.

All employers in the state are required to obtain workers' compensation insurance. Currently, the law gives the employee free choice of the provider to be used for care. A new and revised law was recently enacted. In 18 months, responsibility for choosing a provider to care for an injured worker is being shifted to the employer. Under this new law, employers will select the medical provider that will treat an injured worker.

This new law also changes the appeal process established for the workers' compensation system. The appeal process will continue to flow through the circuit court and the state Supreme Court, and employees will still have 30 days from the time of the injury to initiate an appeal. Questions reviewed under the new appeals process, however, will pertain to law only and do not permit a jury trial. The old system permitted reviews of law and fact and permitted a jury trial.

This new workers' compensation legislation is felt by most people to be a tightening up of the system from the perspective of the employee. It will also increase competition for workers' compensation business among providers. Many in the state will be watching the new system carefully. For example, a recent newspaper story from Capital City reported results of a study of the current system that was completed by the Teamsters and Service Workers Unions. The study reported that under the current system, the state's rejection rate of workers' compensation claims was extremely high and had been increasing for at least the past four years. Rejected claims are not paid by the state. Rejected claims are the responsibility of the employees' regular health insurance plans, which often include deductibles and copayments. The unions identified these shifts of coverage from the state workers' compensation system to the employee and employer as a major source of increasing health insurance expenses. The impact of the new law is unknown.

At its recent annual meeting the State Medical Society endorsed statewide tort reform, similar to the systems adopted in Texas in 2003. The State Medical Society recommends limiting noneconomic damages to $700,000. Policy action committees have been established in each county to work with state representatives to implement this revised system.

Capital City Medical Center has recently purchased a five-year land option in Jasper (near the new interstate) and indicated that it is considering establishing a medical office building with select ancillary services for its physicians. It expects to announce its formal plans in the next 18 to 24 months.

Town	1989	1994	1999	2004	2009	2014
Middleboro	44,590	45,460	45,861	46,995	47,364	47,590
Jasper	28,452	31,560	39,871	42,657	46,902	49,247
Harris City	11,950	12,009	12,203	12,953	12,951	12,904
Statesville	10,840	11,788	11,750	11,790	12,750	14,350
Mifflenville	10,310	10,325	10,623	10,945	10,952	11,240
Carterville	2,310	2,356	2,367	2,145	2,378	2,066
Minortown	2,077	2,160	2,163	2,190	2,056	2,103
Boalsburg	1,759	1,790	1,885	1,893	1,891	1,935
Total	**112,288**	**117,448**	**126,723**	**131,568**	**137,244**	**141,435**
Other Towns Outside Hillsboro County						
Capital City	110,450	120,450	155,340	160,230	163,440	177,560
University Town	78,990	81,044	81,370	83,560	84,500	85,840

TABLE 1.1
Hillsboro County Population: 1989-2014

(This table can also be found online at ache.org/books/Middleboro.)

Town	Population	White	Black	Other
Middleboro	47,590	34,891	9,234	3,465
Jasper	49,247	46,879	1,367	1,001
Harris City	12,904	12,256	130	518
Statesville	14,350	14,078	16	256
Mifflenville	11,240	10,855	301	84
Carterville	2,066	1,958	7	101
Minortown	2,103	2,099	0	4
Boalsburg	1,935	1,924	6	5
Total	**141,435**	**124,940**	**11,061**	**5,434**

TABLE 1.2
Hillsboro County Population by Race—2014 Data Estimate

TABLE 1.3

Age Profile for Hillsboro County by Sex for 2014

Town	TOTAL	Under 5	5–14	15–24	25–44	45–64	65–74	75+
				Age Profiles				
Middleboro	47,590	3,165	5,850	5,378	15,067	9,007	4,703	4,420
Male	22,562	1,690	3,097	2,278	7,289	4,438	2,260	1,510
Female	25,028	1,475	2,753	3,100	7,778	4,569	2,443	2,910
Jasper	49,247	4,128	6,567	6,228	21,420	7,011	3,203	690
Male	24,702	1,904	3,256	3,086	11,349	3,531	1,456	120
Female	24,545	2,224	3,311	3,142	10,071	3,480	1,747	570
Harris City	12,904	812	1,519	1,567	2,883	4,224	976	923
Male	6,314	412	795	796	1,679	2,090	420	122
Female	6,590	400	724	771	1,204	2,134	556	801
Statesville	14,350	1,176	2,168	2,881	3,876	3,367	314	568
Male	7,142	590	1,077	1,445	1,973	1,707	155	195
Female	7,208	586	1,091	1,436	1,903	1,660	159	373
Mifflenville	11,240	1,050	1,030	1,780	2,175	3,337	961	907
Male	5,628	512	577	886	1,156	1,890	426	181
Female	5,612	538	453	894	1,019	1,447	535	726
Carterville	2,066	118	120	442	297	438	406	245
Male	888	56	57	208	147	188	155	77
Female	1,178	62	63	234	150	250	251	168
Minortown	2,103	101	139	268	407	487	390	311
Male	982	50	69	139	213	268	192	51
Female	1,121	51	70	129	194	219	198	260
Boalsburg	1,935	31	75	175	207	500	525	422
Male	911	13	36	77	110	249	260	166
Female	1,024	18	39	98	97	251	265	256
Total	141,435	10,581	17,468	18,719	46,332	28,371	11,478	8,486
Male	69,129	5,227	8,964	8,915	23,916	14,361	5,324	2,422
Female	72,306	5,354	8,504	9,804	22,416	14,010	6,154	6,064

(This table can also be found online at ache.org/books/Middleboro.)

TABLE 1.4
Distance (miles) Between Communities in Hillsboro County

Town	Boalsburg	Carterville	Harris City	Jasper	Middleboro	Mifflenville	Minortown	Statesville
Boalsburg	0	23	9	37	20	16	18	35
Carterville		0	18	28	11	7	13	15
Harris City			0	32	15	11	17	30
Jasper				0	23	21	27	6
Middleboro					0	4	10	23
Mifflenville						0	6	19
Minortown							0	25
Statesville								0
Towns Outside Hillsboro County								
Capital City	61	52	60	22	45	49	55	25
University Town	90	81	85	93	70	74	80	93

TABLE 1.5
Hillsboro County Health Insurance Profile, 2013-2014 (Percent of Total)

Percent of Coverage	Not covered any time during the year	Covered by employment-based insurance	Covered by own employment-based insurance (self-employed)	Covered by Medicaid and private insurance	Covered by Medicare and private insurance	Covered by Medicare and Medicaid
All Residents	**19.3**	**55.1**	**28.6**	**2.8**	**7.5**	**2.1**
Employer size, workers aged 18–64						
Fewer than 25 employees	32.7	50.6	12.4	1.0	0.2	0.2
25–99 employees	25.6	70.5	8.3	1.5	0.1	0
100–499 employees	14.9	76.6	5.6	1.5	0.2	0.3
500-999 employees	13.6	78.8	0.0	0.7	0.2	0.3
1,000+ employees	0.0	0.0	0.0	0.0	0.0	0.0
Household income						
Less than $25,000	28.3	7.3	8.2	0.00	8.1	0.00
$25,000 to $49,999	22.8	43.4	23.6	0.00	15.4	0.00
$50,000 to $74,999	13.2	64.1	30.5	0.00	7.5	0.00
$75,000 or more	9.3	79.5	39.4	0.00	5.7	0.00

NOTE: Percentages may exceed 100% depending on changes during the year of study and multiple coverage. (This table can also be found online at ache.org/books/Middleboro.)

Employer	Fee for Service (FFS)		Managed Care (MC)		Employee Contribution	
	Deductible ($)	Copay (%)	Deductible ($)	Copay (%) Per MD Visit	FFS (%)	MC (%)
Carlstead Rayon	500	80/20			40	40
PPO			300	80/20		
HMO			0	15		
River Industries	1,000	70/30	No Plan		45	NA
Master Tractor	375	70/30				
PPO			350	75/25	30	30
HMO			No Plan			
US Parts	400	80/20				
PPO			300	85/15	25	20
HMO			0	15		
National Yearbooks	750	75/25			30	30
PPO			350	80/20		
HMO			0	10		
Office Pro	1,000	60/40	No Plan		35	NA
Chicken Farms, Inc.	1,000	75/25	300	85/15	25	30
Middleboro Trust	500	80/20			25	25
PPO			500	85/15		
HMO			0	5		

TABLE 1.6

Health Insurance Benefits of Major Area Employers

NOTES: Deductibles shown are for family coverage.

Mental health coverage: State law mandates mental health coverage in any insurance plan with more than 25 participants. The plan must include 30 hours of coverage for outpatient visits and 20 days for inpatient coverage.

TABLE 1.7

Hillsboro County
Estimated
Health Insurance
Coverage (percent
of total)

Coverage	1989	1994	1999	2004	2009	2014
No insurance	12.3	12.5	12.9	14.5	19.1	19.3
Medicaid	11.6	12.7	15.1	15.2	16.3	19.2
Any private plan	66.8	63.6	59.6	58.4	56.3	55.1
Medicare	13.2	14.3	13.7	14.1	14.9	15.0
Military healthcare	1.3	2.0	2.5	2.8	2.4	2.4

NOTE: Total insured and totals may exceed 100% because of multiple coverages.

TABLE 1.8

Estimated Number
of Active Cases in
Hillsboro County,
2009 and 2014

	2009	2014
Sexually transmitted diseases		
Chlamydia	453	455
Gonorrhea	92	103
Syphilis	19	17
Cancer		
Breast	NA	1,301
Colon/rectum	NA	493
Kidney and renal pelvis	NA	121
Leukemia	NA	143
Lung and bronchus	NA	168
Melanoma	NA	312
Non-Hodgkin lymphoma	NA	120
Prostate	NA	956
Urinary bladder	NA	188

	2014	2009	2004
AIDS cases	**Rate per 100,000 population, all ages**		
Hillsboro County	6.9	7.2	7.8
Capital City	8.4	9.3	11.2
Statewide	12.5	13.4	14.5
AIDS cases	**Rate per 100,000 population, adults and adolescents**		
Hillsboro County	7.0	7.4	8.2
Capital City	8.5	9.6	11.5
Statewide	15.2	16.0	18.3
AIDS case rates	**adults and adolescents, rates per 100,000 by sex**		
Hillsboro County			
Male	20.9	23.5	17.2
Female	6.3	7.9	5.4
Capital City			
Male	22.9	24.0	21.3
Female	7.7	7.7	7.9
Statewide			
Male	22.9	26.3	30.1
Female	7.7	6.7	6.7
AIDS cases	**Distribution of persons estimated to be living with AIDS (%)**		
Hillsboro County			
White	70.9	71.2	67.3
Black	18.8	19.3	20.3
Hispanic	4.4	4.4	6.2
Other	5.9	5.1	6.2
Capital City			
White	48.2	40.3	35.5
Black	35.7	40.7	44.5
Hispanic	13.4	16.7	17.3
Other	2.7	2.3	2.7

TABLE 1.9

HIV and AIDS in Capital City and Hillsboro County, 2004–2014

(continued)

TABLE 1.9
HIV and AIDS in
Capital City and
Hillsboro County,
2004–2014
(continued)

	2014	2009	2004
Statewide			
White	34.1	30.2	28.4
Black	42.7	44	44.3
Hispanic	20.9	23.2	25.2
Other	2.3	2.6	2.1
HIV	**Age-adjusted death rate per 100,000 for HIV**		
Hillsboro County	1.1	1.2	1.1
Capital City	3.8	3.2	3.2
Statewide	4.2	4.6	4.8
HIV	**Estimated rate per 100,000 for persons living with HIV infections (not AIDS)**		
Hillsboro County	22.7	21.3	24.3
Capital City	34.5	36.7	39.5
Statewide	51.7	48.3	50.2

HIV—2014	**Rates per 100,000 of new HIV infections in adults and adolescents**		
	Males	**Females**	**Total**
Hillsboro County			
White	10.5	2.2	7.1
Black	80.7	21.7	51.9
Hispanic	31.2	6.3	19.2
Capital City			
White	13.5	4.1	9.1
Black	112.4	50.9	82.7
Hispanic	47.5	13.0	30.7
Statewide			
White	19.6	3.9	11.5
Black	115.7	55.7	83.7
Hispanic	43.8	14.4	29.3

(This table can also be found online at ache.org/books/Middleboro.)

	2014	2009
	Cases	**Cases**
Hillsboro County		
45–64	3,093	2,480
65–74	2,233	1,890
75+	1,326	1,268
Total	7,826	6,632
Capital City		
45–64	3,811	3,396
65–74	2,806	2,590
75+	1,597	2,417
Total	9,625	9,886
	Deaths	**Deaths**
Hillsboro County		
Males	18	20
Females	15	13
Total	33	33
Capital City		
Males	25	18
Females	20	16
Total	45	34
	Deaths	**Deaths**
Hillsboro County		
White	25	20
Black	5	10
Other	3	3
Capital City		
White	21	24
Black	18	16
Other	6	4

TABLE 1.10

Diabetes in Capital City and Hillsboro County by Age, Gender, and Race: 2014 and 2009

NOTE: Discrepancy in totals because of cases under age 45

TABLE 1.11
BRFSS Data

	Hillsboro County	Capital City
Alcohol consumption		
Adults who have had at least one drink of alcohol within the past 30 days	38.2%	58.5%
Heavy drinkers (adult men having more than two drinks per day and adult women having more than one drink per day)	2.5%	5.1%
Binge drinkers (adults having five or more drinks on one occasion)	8.4%	14.2%
Arthritis		
Adults who have been told they have arthritis	29.3%	24.0%
Asthma		
Adults who have been told they currently have asthma	10.5%	9.0%
Adults who have ever been told they have asthma	13.8%	13.2%
Cardiovascular disease		
Adults who have been told they had a heart attack (myocardial infarction)	4.3%	4.3%
Adults who have been told they had angina or coronary heart disease	5.3%	4.7%
Adults who have been told they had a stroke	3.3%	2.7%
Cholesterol awareness		
Adults who have had their blood cholesterol checked within the last five years	65.3%	71.2%
Adults who have ever had their blood cholesterol checked	82.4%	73.2%
Adults who have had their blood cholesterol checked and have been told it was high	56.6%	40.4%
Colorectal cancer		
Adults aged 50+ who have had a blood stool test within the past two years.	15.6%	21.3%
Adults aged 50+ who have had a sigmoidoscopy or colonoscopy	51.0%	68.0%

(continued)

TABLE **1.11**
BRFSS Data
(continued)

	Hillsboro County	Capital City
Diabetes		
Have you ever been told by a doctor that you have diabetes?- No	93.5%	83.4%
Disability		
Adults with health problems that requires the use of special equipment	8.3%	21.2%
Adults who are limited in any activities because of physical, mental, or emotional problem	12.3%	17.4%
Exercise		
Participated in any physical activities in the past month	80.3%	70.2%
Fruits and vegetables		
Consumed fruits and vegetables five or more times per day	29.4%	19.4%
Healthcare access/coverage		
Access to healthcare coverage	78.2%	72.3%
Health status		
Excellent	22.2%	23.4%
Very good	25.5%	37.6%
Good	27.0%	30.5%
Fair	14.5%	6.3%
Poor	10.8%	2.2%
Hypertension awareness		
Adults who have been told they have high blood pressure	34.5%	26.3%
Immunization status		
Adults aged 65+ who had a flu shot within the past year	43.4%	54.2%
Adults aged 65+ who have ever had a pneumonia vaccination	23.5%	43.4%
Oral health		
Adults aged 65+ who have had all their natural teeth extracted	18.9%	13.4%

(continued)

TABLE 1.11
BRFSS Data
(continued)

	Hillsboro County	Capital City
Adults that have had any permanent teeth extracted	64.2%	58.3%
Visited the dentist or dental clinic within the past year for any reason	61.3%	70.8%
Physical activity		
Adults with 30+ minutes of moderate physical activity five or more days per week, or vigorous physical activity for 20+ minutes three or more days per week	52.2%	40.4%
Adults with 20+ minutes of vigorous physical activity three or more days per week	30.4%	28.9%
Prostate cancer		
Men aged 40+ who have had a PSA test within the past two years	59.3%	53.3%
Women's health		
Women aged 50+ who have had a mammogram within the past two years	77.1%	82.4%
Women aged 18+ who have had a pap test within the past three years	77.5%	82.8%
Women aged 40+ who have had a mammogram with the past two years	65.8%	70.3%
Tobacco use		
Four-Level Smoking Status		
Daily	24.5%	21.4%
Some days	7.5%	6.7%
Former smoker	14.0%	20.2%
Never smoked	54.0%	51.7%
Adults who are current smokers	32.0%	28.1%
Demographics		
Age		
18–24 years	9.0%	12.5%
25–34 years	19.5%	16.5%

(continued)

	Hillsboro County	Capital City
35–44 years	20.4%	21.5%
45–54 years	23.5%	19.5%
55–64 years	8.8%	14.0%
65+ years	18.8%	16.0%
Race/ethnicity		
White	84.0%	78.0%
Black	10.0%	12.5%
Hispanic	4.0%	5.5%
Other	1.0%	2.0%
Multiracial	1.0%	2.0%
Marital status		
Married	73.0%	65.0%
Divorced	6.0%	10.3%
Widowed	8.8%	7.3%
Separated	1.3%	1.0%
Never married	10.5%	14.2%
Partnered	0.4%	2.2%
Children in household		
None	50.1%	63.2%
One	16.9%	17.2%
Two	22.5%	15.2%
Three	5.5%	3.1%
Four	3.2%	1.0%
Five or more	1.8%	0.3%
Highest grade in school		
Less than high school	10.2%	11.3%
Diploma or GED	44.5%	34.5%

TABLE 1.11
BRFSS Data
(continued)

(continued)

TABLE 1.11
BRFSS Data
(continued)

	Hillsboro County	Capital City
Some post-high school	18.2%	28.3%
College+	27.1%	25.9%
Employment		
Employed	54.3%	48.2%
Self-employed	10.5%	7.5%
Unemployed more than 1 year	0.4%	2.3%
Unemployed less than 1 year	1.2%	2.9%
Homemaker	9.3%	6.9%
Student	4.0%	4.8%
Retired	17.3%	22.2%
Unable to work	3.0%	5.2%
Household income		
Less than $15,000	12.4%	14.8%
$15,000–$24,999	18.3%	11.3%
$25,000–$34,999	10.2%	10.8%
$35,000–$49,999	18.9%	11.8%
$50,000+	40.2%	51.3%
Gender		
Male	49.5%	46.3%
Female	51.5%	53.7%
Weight classification		
Neither overweight not obese (BMI below 24.9)	33.2%	29.0%
Overweight (BMI 25.0–29.9)	38.8%	39.0%
Obese (BMI 30.0–99.8)	28.0%	32.0%
Sample size	860	1,245

NOTE: BRFSS is the Behavioral Risk Factor Surveillance System designed by the Centers for Disease Control and Prevention (CDC). Reported percentages are based on cell sizes > 50.

	Percent of Population 18+ Years of Age
Total population with asthma	10.5
Gender	
Male	6.4
Female	14.3
Age	
18–34	11.7
35–64	10.8
65+	7.6
Household income	
<$25,000	15.8
$25,000+	9.3
Education level	
Less than high school	18.3
At least high school/GED	10.0
Employment status	
Employed	9.4
Unemployed	12.7
Unable to work	27.5
Homemaker/student	14.0
Retired	7.9
Insurance	
Employer	9.5
Medicare	10.1
Medicaid	35.2
Other	9.8
No insurance	11.6

TABLE 1.12
Prevalence of Asthma in Hillsboro County, 2014

	Note	2020 Goals	State 2010
Access to health services			
Percent of adults under 65 with health insurance		100.0	84.0
Percent of adults 18–64 with specific source of ongoing care		89.0	72.0
Percent of adults 65+ with specific source of ongoing care		100.0	74.0
Arthritis, osteoporosis, and chronic back conditions			
Percent of adults with doctor-diagnosed arthritis whose usual activities are limited in any way by arthritis		35.5	26.0
Percent of adults 18–64 diagnosed with arthritis who are unemployed or unable to work		31.5	22.0
Hospitalization rate for hip fracture among females 65+	1	741.2	819.2
Hospitalization rate for hip fracture among males 65+	1	418.4	490.5
Cancer			
Lung cancer death rate	1	48.5	52.4
Breast cancer death rate	1	20.6	25.0
Cervical cancer death rate	1	2.2	2.6
Colorectal cancer death rate	1	14.5	19.4
Oropharyngeal cancer death rate	1	2.3	2.2
Prostate cancer death rate	1	21.2	27.1
Melanoma (skin) cancer death rate	1	2.4	2.7
Percent of women 21–65 who have received cervical cancer screening based on the most recent guidelines		93.0	81.2
Percent of adults 50+ who received a fecal occult blood test for colorectal cancer within the past 2 years	1	17.0	17.0
Percent of adults aged 50 who ever received a sigmoidscopy for colorectal cancer	1	72.0	68.0
Percent of women 50–74 with a mammogram in last 2 years	1	81.1	70.0
Chronic kidney disease			
End-stage renal disease incidence rate	2	318.5	358.6
Diabetes			
Percent of adults with diabetes who have an annual foot examination.	1	74.8	66.1
Percent of adults with diabetes who have an annual dilated eye examination	1	58.7	68.3
Percent of adults with diabetes who have a glycosylated hemoglobin measurement at least twice a year.	1	71.7	66.4
Percent of adults with diabetes who perform self-blood-glucose monitoring at least once daily.	1	70.4	55.8
Percent of adults diagnosed with diabetes who have attended class in managing diabetes.	1	62.5	60.0
Environmental health			
Number of days the Air Quality Index exceeds 100.		10.0	26.0
Percent of persons receiving safe drinking water from community water systems.		91.0	90.0

(continued)

	Note	2020 Goals	State 2010
Waterborne disease outbreaks from community water systems		0.0	0.0
State monitors environment-related diseases		Yes	Yes
Family planning			
Pregnancy rate among adolescent females 15–17	3	36.2	23.6
Food safety			
Campylobacter species incidence	4	8.5	12.8
Shigs toxin-producing E-coli	4	0.6	1.2
Salmonella incidence rate	4	11.4	13.7
Outbreaks of infections associated with beef		0.0	0.0
Hearing and other sensory or communication disorders			
Percent of infants (with possible hearing loss) who receive audiologic evaluation by age 3 months		72.6	70.9
Health communication			
Percent of persons with access to Internet		80	80
Heart disease and stroke			
Coronary heart disease death rate	1	100.8	153.1
Stroke death rate	1	33.8	47.9
Percent of adults aged 20 and older ever told blood pressure was high		10% decrease	29.0
Percent of adults who had their blood cholesterol checked within the last 5 years		82.1	75.0
Hospitalization rate for heart failure as the principal diagnosis (65–74)	5	8.8	12.4
Hospitalization rate for heart failure as the principal diagnosis (75–84)	5	20.2	30.1
Hospitalization rate for heart failure as the principal diagnosis (85+)	5	38.6	67.2
HIV			
AIDS incidence rate (persons aged 13+)	6	13.0	14.2
Number of new AIDS cases among men aged 13+ who have sex with men		10% decrease	438.0
Number of new AIDS cases among persons aged 13+ who inject drugs		10% decrease	353.0
Number of new cases of perinatally acquired AIDS		10% decrease	4.0
HIV disease death rate	1	3.3	2.9
Percent of persons aged 25–44 with tuberculosis who have been tested for HIV		71.5	79.0
Percent of unmarried sexually active women (18–44) who use condoms (to prevent pregnancy)		38.0	21.5
Percent of unmarried sexually active men (18–44) who use condoms (to prevent pregnancy)		60.7	n/a

TABLE 1.13

Healthy People 2020 National Goals and 2010 State Statistics (continued)

(continued)

	Note	2020 Goals	State 2010
Immunization and infectious disease			
Number of new reported cases of vaccine-preventable diseases: Pertussis (under 1)		Reduce	82.0
Number of new reported cases of vaccine-preventable diseases: Pertussis (11–18)		Reduce	140.0
Number of new reported cases of vaccine-preventable diseases: Varicella/chicken pox (under 18)		Reduce	4,869.0
Meningococcal disease incidence rate	1	0.3	0.5
Percent of vaccination coverage levels of 4 doses diphtheria-tetanus-acellular pertussis (children 19–35 months)		90.0	87.8
Percent of vaccination coverage levels for 3 doses Haemophilus influenza type b (children 19–35 months)		90.0	95.0
Percent of vaccination coverage levels for 3 doses hepatitis B (children 19–35 months)		90.0	92.4
Percent of vaccination coverage levels for 1 dose measles-mumps-rubella (children 19–35 months)		90.0	94.0
Percent of vaccination coverage levels for 3 doses polio (children 19–35 months)		90.0	93.9
Percent of vaccination coverage levels for 1 dose varicella (children 19–35 months)		90.0	88.9
Percent of vaccination coverage levels for 4 doses pneumococcal conjugate (children 19–35 months)		90.0	75.8
Percent of fully immunized children (19–35 months)		80.0	68.3
Percent of adults 18–64 with flu shot in past year		80.0	31.2
Percent of adults 65+ with flu shot in past year		90.0	72.2
Percent of adults 65+ ever vaccinated against pneumococcal disease		90.0	69.0
Percent of adults 18–64 who ever had vaccination against pneumococcal disease		10% increase	15.2
Percent of public health providers who had vaccination coverage levels among children in their practice population measured within the last year		50.0	80.0
Percent of children under 6 who participate in population-based immunization registries		10% increase	17.0
Hepatitis A incidence rate	1	0.3	0.5
Hepatitis B incidence rate (persons 19+)	1	1.5	1.1
Hepatitis C incidence rate	1	0.2	0.4
Tuberculosis incidence rate	1	1.0	2.7
Percent of tuberculosis patients who complete curative therapy within 12 months		93.0	74.0
Percent of persons with latent tuberculosis infection who complete a course of treatment		79.0	41.0

(continued)

	Note	2020 Goals	State 2010
Injury and violence prevention			
Hospitalization rate for nonfatal traumatic brain injuries	1	10% decrease	39.6
Hospitalization rate for nonfatal spinal cord injuries	1	3.2	5.8
State-level child fatality review of external causes for children 17 and under.		Yes	Yes
Statewide emergency department surveillance system that collects data on external causes of injury.		Yes	No
State collects data on external causes of injury through hospital discharge data systems.		Yes	Yes
Poisoning death rate	1	13.1	15.3
Unintentional injury death rate	1	36.0	39.4
Motor vehicle crash death rate	1	12.4	12.2
Motor vehicle crash death rate	7	1.2	1.5
Percent of adults using safety belts		92.4	75.1
Pedestrian death rate	1	1.3	1.4
State law requiring bicycle helmets for riders under 18		Yes	No
Accidental falls death rate	1	7.0	6.5
Unintentional suffocation death rate	1	1.7	2.3
Drowning death rate	1	1.1	0.9
Residential fire death rate	1	0.9	1.2
Homicide rate	1	5.5	6.3
Firearm-related death rate	1	9.2	10.8
Weapon possession among adolescents on school property	8	10% decrease	1.8
Child maltreatment fatality rate	9	2.1	1.1
Maltreatment of children under 18	9	8.5	8.0
Maternal, infant, and child health			
Fetal mortality rate (20+ weeks gestation)	10	5.6	6.0
Perinatal mortality rate (fetal and infant mortality rate during perinatal period)	10	5.9	7.1
Infant mortality rate (under 1 year of age)	10	6.0	7.2
Neonatal mortality rate (0–27 days of age)	10	4.1	5.1
Postneonatal mortality rate (28–364 days of age)	10	2.0	2.1
Infant mortality rate for birth defects	10	1.3	1.3
Infant mortality rate for congenital heart defects	10	0.3	0.4
Infant mortality rate for sudden infant death syndrome	10	0.5	0.4
Child 1–4 death rate	11	25.7	26.1
Child 5–9 death rate	11	12.3	13.1

TABLE 1.13

Healthy People 2020 National Goals and 2010 State Statistics (continued)

(continued)

TABLE 1.13

Healthy People
2020 National
Goals and 2010
State Statistics
(continued)

	Note	2020 Goals	State 2010
Adolescent 10–14 death rate	11	15.2	16.6
Adolescent 15–19 death rate	11	55.7	57.4
Young adult 20–24 death rate	11	88.5	103.5
Maternal mortality rate	10	11.4	10.3
Rate of maternal complications during hospitalized labor and delivery.	12	28.0	35.1
Percent of low-risk first-time mothers giving birth by cesarean		23.9	27.5
Percent of low-risk women giving birth by cesarean with a prior cesarean birth		81.7	86.0
Percent of infants born at low birth weight		7.8	8.5
Percent of infants born at very low birth weight		1.4	1.6
Percent of preterm live births		11.4	10.2
Percent of live births at 34–36 weeks of gestation		8.1	7.3
Percent of live births at 32–33 weeks of gestation		1.4	1.3
Percent of live births at less than 32 weeks of gestation		1.8	1.8
Percent births to mothers beginning prenatal care in first trimester		77.9	71.5
Percent live births to mothers who received early and adequate prenatal care		77.6	66.3
Percent of live births to mothers who did not smoke during pregnancy		98.6	82.4
Percent of mothers who breastfeed their babies		81.9	64.6
All newborns screened at birth for conditions as mandated by state programs		Yes	Yes
Percent of very low birth weight infants born at Level III hospitals		83.7	83.7
Mental health and mental disorders			
Suicide rate	1	10.2	10.7
Nutrition and weight status			
Percent of healthy weight adults (age 20+)		33.9	34.2
Percent of obese adults (age 20+)		30.6	29.2
Percent of children grades K–6 who are obese		15.7	17.3
Percent of children grades 7–12 who are obese		16.1	17.2
Occupational safety and health			
Work-related injury death rate for all industries (aged 16+)	13	3.6	3.2
Work-related injury death rate for construction industry (aged 16+)	13	9.7	7.9
Work-related injury death rate for transportation and warehousing industry (aged 16+)	13	14.8	10.7
Number of pneumoconiosis deaths (aged 15+)		10% decrease	329.0
Work-related homicides (aged 16+)		10 less	29.0

(continued)

	Note	2020 Goals	State 2010
Oral health			
Percent of adults 45–64 who ever had a permanent tooth extracted due to dental caries or periodontal disease.		68.8	55.5
Percent of oral and pharyngeal cancers detected at the earliest stage		35.8	31.7
Percent of adults who have visited a dentist in the past year, persons 18+ and 65+		10% increase	70.2, 65.3
Percent of population served by optimally fluoridated community water systems		79.6	46.0
State has a system for referring infants/children with cleft lips, cleft palates, and other craniofacial anomalies to rehabilitative teams.		Yes	Yes
State has an oral and craniofacial state-based surveillance system		Yes	No
State has an effective public dental health program directed by a dental professional with public health training.		Yes	Yes
Physical activity			
Percent adults who engage in no leisure-time physical activity.		32.6	23.2
Percent adults who engage in vigorous or moderate physical activity		10% increase	51.2
Public health infrastucture			
State public health agency provides epidemiology services to support essential public health services		Yes	Yes
State has a health improvement plan		Yes	Yes
Respiratory disease			
Asthma death rate (under 35)	14	10% decrease	4.5
Asthma death rate (35–64)	14	6.0	12.6
Asthma death rate (65+)	14	22.9	37.8
Hospitalization rate for asthma (under 5)	15	18.1	47.1
Hospitalization rate for asthma (5–64)	15	8.6	14.9
Hospitalization rate for asthma (65+)	15	20.3	28.2
State asthma surveillance system for tracking asthma cases, illness, and disability.		Yes	No
Death rate due to chronic obstructive pulmonary disease among adults 45+	1	98.5	109.7
Sexually transmitted disease			
Gonorrhea incidence rate among females 15–44	1	251.9	225.4
Gonorrhea incidence rate among males 15–44	1	194.8	164.2
Incidence rate of primary and secondary syphilis among females	1	1.3	0.5
Incidence rate of primary and secondary syphilis among males	1	6.7	3.8

TABLE 1.13

Healthy People 2020 National Goals and 2010 State Statistics (continued)

(continued)

TABLE 1.13

Healthy People
2020 National
Goals and 2010
State Statistics
(continued)

	Note	2020 Goals	State 2010
Substance abuse			
Percent of high school seniors who never used any alcoholic beverages		30.5	17.3
Percent of 8th graders who disapprove of drinking alcohol regularly		86.4	87.2
Percent of 10th graders who disapprove of drinking alcohol regularly		85.4	61.3
Percent of 12th graders who disapprove of drinking alcohol regularly		77.6	48.2
Percent of 8th graders who said they would never use marijuana		82.8	84.2
Percent of 10th graders who said they would never use marijuana		66.1	65.4
Percent of 12th graders who said they would never use marijuana		60.3	50.5
Cirrhosis death rate	1	8.2	7.2
Drug-induced death rate	1	11.3	14.6
Percent of high school seniors who engaged in binge drinking in past two weeks		22.7	34.4
Tobacco use			
Percent of adults who smoke cigarettes		12.0	22.2
Percent of adults who use smokeless (spit) tobacco		0.3	3.1
Percent of adults who smoke cigars		0.2	7.1
Percent of students in grades 9–12 who used tobacco products in past month		21.0	25.3
Percent of students in grades 9–12 who smoked cigarettes in past month		16.0	17.3
Percent of students in grades 9–12 who used smokeless (spit) tobacco in past month		6.9	6.2
Percent of students in grades 9–12 who used cigars in past month		8.0	10.2
Percent of adult smokers who attempted to quit smoking		80.0	57.4
Percent smoke cessation during first trimester of pregnancy		30.0	24.8
Percent of students in grades 9–12 who tried to quit smoking		64.0	66.8
State has smoke-free indoor air laws that prohibit smoking		Yes	Mixed

NOTES

1. per 100,000
2. per 1,000,000
3. per 1,000 women 15–17
4. cases per 100,000
5. per 1,000 by age group
6. per 100,000 ages 13+
7. per million miles traveled
8. per 1,000 students
9. per 100,000 children under 18
10. per 1,000 live births
11. per 100,000 in age group
12. per 100 deliveries
13. per 100,000 workers 16+
14. per 1,000,000
15. per 10,000

Town	Population	Hospital Discharges	Patient Days			
			Total	Webster Hospital (WH)	Middleboro Community Hospital (MCH)	Other
Jasper						
2014	49,247	5,352	24,084	3,013	17,100	3,971
2009	46,902	4,878	22,926	3,078	17,664	2,184
2004	42,657	4,795	24,453	3,105	19,825	1,523
Middleboro						
2014	47,590	6,201	35,346	7,076	27,830	440
2009	47,364	6,394	33,889	4,850	28,185	854
2004	46,995	7,364	43,448	4,445	38,143	860
Statesville						
2014	14,350	1,530	7,191	3,020	4,056	115
2009	12,750	1,469	7,938	3,175	4,673	90
2004	11,790	1,455	8,293	3,375	4,846	72
Harris City						
2014	12,904	1,730	8,996	6,743	2,020	233
2009	12,951	1,756	12,117	9,866	2,006	245
2004	12,953	1,886	12,447	7,856	4,360	231
Mifflenville						
2014	11,240	1,456	7,280	2,839	4,288	153
2009	10,952	1,687	8,939	3,320	5,475	144
2004	10,945	1,795	10,411	2,003	8,230	178
Carterville						
2014	2,066	330	1,716	596	1,077	43
2009	2,378	338	1,891	702	1,177	12
2004	2,145	332	2,095	723	1,283	89
Minortown						
2014	2,103	420	2,408	601	1,796	11
2009	2,056	317	1,963	508	1,448	7
2004	2,190	382	2,446	468	1,962	16
Boalsburg						
2014	1,935	220	1,217	681	513	23
2009	1,891	236	1,395	747	608	40
2004	1,893	254	1,547	707	761	79
Hillsboro County Totals						
2014	141,435	17,239	88,238	24,569	58,680	4,989
2009	137,244	17,075	91,058	26,246	61,236	3,576
2004	131,568	18,263	105,140	22,682	79,410	3,048

TABLE 1.14

Hospital Discharges and Patient Days

(continued)

TABLE 1.14

Hospital
Discharges and
Patient Days
(continued)

Town	Population	Hospital Discharges	Patient Days			
			Total	Webster Hospital (WH)	Middleboro Community Hospital (MCH)	Other
Noncounty Residents						
2014	n/a	32	176	86	90	
2009	n/a	24	128	45	83	
2004	n/a	21	124	44	80	
Total						
2014			88,414	24,655	58,770	4,989
2009			91,186	26,291	61,319	3,576
2004			105,264	22,726	79,490	3,048
2014 Hospital Discharges by Town and Hospital						
		Total Discharges		WH	MCH	Other
	Jasper		5,352	685	3,450	1,217
	Middleboro		6,201	1,505	4,613	83
	Statesville		1,530	655	850	25
	Harris City		1,730	1,386	304	40
	Mifflenville		1,456	516	910	30
	Carterville		330	118	199	13
	Minortown		420	104	314	2
	Boalsburg		220	126	90	4
		Total Discharges	17,239	5,095	10,730	1,414
		Operating Beds		95	240	

	Total	MCH	WH	Other
General and family practice	38	5	26	7
Middleboro	9	0	9	0
Jasper	10	0	4	6
Harris City	3	0	3	0
Statesville	3	1	1	1
Mifflenville	6	1	5	0
Carterville	2	1	1	0
Minortown	3	1	2	0
Boalsburg	2	1	1	0
Internal medicine	47	33	2	12
Middleboro	12	10	2	0
Jasper	22	10	0	12
Harris City	2	2	0	0
Statesville	2	2	0	0
Mifflenville	4	4	0	0
Carterville	2	2	0	0
Minortown	2	2	0	0
Boalsburg	1	1	0	0
Pediatrics	28	16	4	8
Middleboro	14	10	4	0
Jasper	14	6	0	8
Allergy/immunology	5	3	0	2
Middleboro	2	2	0	0
Jasper	3	1	0	2
Cardiology	8	5	1	2
Middleboro	4	4	0	0
Jasper	4	1	1	2

TABLE 1.15
Physicians by Specialty, by Town, and by Hospital Affiliation, 2014

(continued)

	Total	MCH	WH	Other
Gastroenterology	6	6	0	0
Middleboro	4	4	0	0
Jasper	2	2	0	0
Psychiatry	5	5	0	0
Middleboro	3	3	0	0
Jasper	2	2	0	0
Other medical specialties[1]	17	12	3	2
Middleboro	15	10	3	2
Jasper	2	2	0	0
Orthopedic surgery	12	8	2	2
Middleboro	10	8	2	0
Jasper	2	0	0	2
General surgery	18	12	4	2
Middleboro	14	10	4	0
Jasper	4	2	0	2
OB/GYN	16	8	6	2
Middleboro	14	8	6	0
Jasper	2	0	0	2
Other[2]	17	16	1	0
Middleboro	17	16	1	0
Jasper	0	0	0	0
Total hospital-based	61	43	18	0
Emergency	20	12	8	0
Anesthesiology	14	10	4	0
Radiology	16	13	3	0
Pathology	11	8	3	0
Total	**278**	**172**	**67**	**39**

NOTES: 1. Includes dermatology, pulmonology, endocrinology, ophthalmology, otolaryngology, pulmonary medicine, and oncology and hemotology. 2. Includes vascular surgery, bariatric surgery, eye surgery, plastic surgery, thoracic surgery, urology, and neurosurgery.

Only includes physicians with active medical staff privileges or who are employed by an accredited hospital.

MCH = Middleboro Community Hospital; WH = Webster Hospital; Other = other hospital, a hospital not located in Hillsboro County

	1989	1994	1999	2004	2009	2014
Live births	1,282	1,746	1,945	2,205	2,678	2,935
Deaths (except fetal)	833	890	967	1,085	1,210	1,236
Infant deaths	16	13	21	14	14	17
Neonatal deaths[1]	10	12	13	10	8	6
Postneonatal deaths[2]	6	1	8	4	6	11
Maternal deaths	2	1	1	2	1	2
Out-of-wedlock births	140	167	175	216	299	355
Marriages	1,053	977	923	901	1,051	981

TABLE 1.16

Vital Statistics for Hillsboro County

NOTES: 1. Less than 28 days. 2. Within 28 to 365 days.

Cause of Death	Note	1989	1994	1999	2004	2009	2014
Diseases of the heart	A	302	325	361	390	418	401
Malignant neoplasms (cancer)	B	212	221	234	240	245	256
Cerebrovascular diseases	C	57	60	67	73	86	93
Chronic lower respiratory disease	D	32	32	34	34	36	40
All accidents	E	44	45	49	59	70	64
Alzheimer's disease	F	0	10	16	20	26	34
Diabetes mellitus	G	25	22	30	30	33	33
Influenza and pneumonia	H	31	27	31	40	34	30
Nephritis, nephrotic syndrome, and nephrosis	I	16	23	20	18	21	22
Septicemia	J	5	5	6	9	8	14
Intentional self-harm/suicide	K	14	21	18	20	26	24
Chronic liver disease and cirrhosis	L	12	12	14	13	18	12
Renal disease	M	4	4	7	9	7	11
Parkinson's disease	N	2	2	5	3	6	9
Assault and homicide	O	0	2	3	2	1	4
Total leading causes		756	811	895	960	1,035	1,047
All deaths		833	890	967	1,085	1,210	1,236

TABLE 1.17

Resident Deaths by Cause of Death

NOTES: ICD codes

A = I00-I09, I11, I13, 120-151

B = C00-C97

C = I60-I69

D = J40-J47

E = V03, X60-X84, Y87.0

F = G30

G = E10-E14

H = J09-J18

I = N00-N07, N17-N19, N25-N27

J = A40-A41

K = U03, X60-X84, YB7.0

L = K70, K73 - K74

M = I10, I12, I15

N = G29-G21

O = U01-U02, X85-Y09, Y 87.1

TABLE 1.18
Causes of Resident
Death by Age
Groups: 2014,
2009, and 2004

Cause of Death	Total	Under 1	1–4	5–14	15–24	25–44	45–64	65–75	75+
Diseases of the heart									
2014	401	2	0	0	2	14	58	124	201
2009	418	0	0	0	0	11	50	139	218
2004	390	0	0	0	0	9	40	120	221
Malignant neoplasms (cancer)									
2014	256	1	0	1	1	24	38	79	112
2009	245	0	0	2	4	19	24	75	121
2004	240	0	0	0	0	14	31	77	118
Cerebrovascular diseases									
2014	93	0	0	0	1	3	10	26	53
2009	86	0	0	0	0	2	14	23	47
2004	73	0	0	0	0	5	17	16	35
Chronic lower respiratory disease									
2014	40	0	0	0	0	0	13	13	14
2009	36	0	0	0	0	0	11	9	16
2004	34	0	0	0	0	0	12	8	14
All accidents									
2014	64	5	2	9	8	6	7	8	19
2009	70	3	4	4	18	15	12	5	9
2004	59	5	1	2	13	16	8	3	11
Alzheimer's disease									
2014	34	0	0	0	0	0	2	3	29
2009	26	0	0	0	0	0	1	0	25
2004	20	0	0	0	0	0	1	2	17
Diabetes mellitus									
2014	33	0	0	0	0	0	5	12	16
2009	33	0	0	0	0	2	10	12	9
2004	30	0	0	0	0	1	12	12	5
Influenza and pneumonia									
2014	30	1	0	0	0	0	1	12	16
2009	34	1	2	0	0	0	2	8	21
2004	40	0	1	0	0	4	4	9	22
Nephritis, nephrotic syndrome, and nephrosis									
2014	22	0	1	0	1	2	4	5	9
2009	21	0	0	1	2	4	6	2	6
2004	18	0	1	3	3	1	2	2	6
Septicemia									
2014	14	1	0	0	0	0	2	2	9
2009	13	0	0	0	0	0	1	4	8
2004	14	1	0	0	0	0	3	3	7

(continued)

Cause of Death	Total	Under 1	1–4	5–14	15–24	25–44	45–64	65–74	75+
Intentional self-harm/suicide									
2014	24	0	0	0	2	2	9	5	6
2009	26	0	0	4	6	6	4	2	4
2004	20	0	0	3	2	3	6	4	2
Chronic liver disease and cirrhosis									
2014	12	0	0	0	0	0	3	5	4
2009	18	0	0	0	0	0	6	5	7
2004	13	0	0	0	0	1	4	4	4
Total, listed causes									
CY	1,023	10	3	10	15	51	152	294	488
CY-5	1,026	4	6	11	30	59	141	284	491
CY-10	951	6	3	8	18	54	140	260	462
Total, other causes									
CY	213	7	2	2	24	30	32	51	65
CY-5	184	10	6	12	9	34	19	44	50
CY-10	134	9	1	9	7	9	10	40	49
Total, all deaths									
2014	1,236	17	5	12	39	81	184	345	553
2009	1,210	14	12	23	39	93	160	328	541
2004	1,085	15	4	17	25	63	150	300	511

TABLE 1.18

Causes of Resident Death by Age Groups: 2014, 2009, and 2004 (continued)

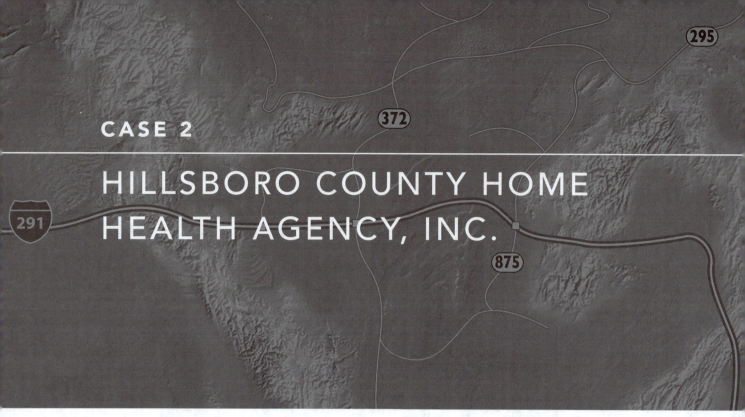

HILLSBORO COUNTY HOME HEALTH AGENCY, INC.

The Hillsboro County Home Health Agency (HCHHA), originally named the Middleboro Home Health Agency, was founded in 1946 as a nonprofit home health agency to provide healthcare services to the area's population. Three years ago, in conjunction with establishing an office in Jasper, the organization changed its name to reflect better its countywide orientation. Today, it is the only Medicare-certified home health agency in Hillsboro County. The Joint Commission also accredits it.

MISSION

"The mission of HCHHA is to serve individuals in their usual environments and is concerned with well people as well as people with illness or disabilities. We strive to prevent disease or to retard its progress and to reduce the ill effects of unavoidable disease. We provide quality nursing and therapeutic care to the noninstitutionalized sick and disabled. We also provide information and encouragement to individuals and families, special groups, and the community as a whole for the promotion of health." (Approved by the board of directors, December 31, 2010.)

GOVERNANCE

Overall responsibility for HCHHA rests with the board of directors. The 21-person board meets monthly to review the status of the corporation. Except as noted the board acts as a committee of the whole. All directors serve for a three-year term and may be reelected by the board. The executive committee nominates individuals for membership on the board. The new board then elects its officers. The election of directors is done by the full board at the June meeting. New directors and officers take their positions beginning July 1. Last year a consultant recommended that the board cease being self-perpetuating and establish mandatory term limits. The board is still considering this concept.

The executive committee (president, vice president, secretary, and treasurer) meets, as needed, with the executive director to resolve special issues and plan board meetings. In April of each year, the executive committee prepares a slate of nominees for new board members. The finance committee meets monthly with the executive director to review the financial status of the corporation. It also reviews and recommends the new annual budget to the full board for approval. The professional advisory committee meets monthly to review issues related to clinical care and quality standards.

Membership on the current board includes Janet Myer, senior vice president at the Middleboro Trust Company. She is currently president of the board of directors and has one year remaining on her third three-year term. She lives in Middleboro. This is her fourth consecutive year as board president. It should be noted that Myer was instrumental in the reorganization of the agency three years ago. David Ruseski, owner of Ruseski Auto Sales in Middleboro and Jasper, is in his second year as vice president of the board. His first three-year term on the board will expire next June, but he has agreed to serve for another three-year term if he is nominated. During 2012 he chaired the finance committee. Ruseski lives in Mifflenville. Mary Steel, JD, is the elected secretary. She maintains her solo law practice in Mifflenville and lives in Middleboro. Steel has been on the board for nine years. Steve Meadows is the elected treasurer. He is the senior partner in the accounting firm of Meadows and Associates in Middleboro. He has served on the board for 14 years. As treasurer, he is a member of the finance committee. He lives in Statesville.

William Bond, vice president of finance at Master Tractor, was elected to his first term on the board two years ago. He chairs the finance committee and has indicated that he will be unable to serve beyond this coming June. He lives in Mifflenville. Martha Logic, JD, is an attorney in the law offices of the Jasper Legal Assistance Clinic and has served on the board for five years. She lives in Jasper. Carl Fisher was elected to the board for his first term three years ago. He is a retired major general from the US Army and is active in the local chapter of the AARP. He maintains farming interests at his family's farm in Boalsburg. Nancy Blau was elected to the board for her first term two years ago. She is a former county commissioner, a member of the regional school board, and a trustee at Webster Hospital. She lives in Middleboro. She serves on the finance committee. Helen Vosper, RN, was reelected to the board four years ago. She was the director of nursing at Middleboro Community Hospital until 2010 and recently retired as director of nursing at Webster Hospital. She lives in Middleboro. Lois Metz, MSW, was elected to the board last July and is serving her first term. She maintains her independent practice as a social worker in Middleboro, where she specializes in marriage and family counseling. She lives in Middleboro. Janet Doe was reelected to the board two years ago. She is a retired registered nurse and the former director of school nursing for public schools in Middleboro. She resides in Middleboro and has been a member of the board for 16 years. Melissa Giles, a recent law school graduate and alumna of the Middleboro school system, was elected to the board last year. She is currently a legislative aide to US Representative James Giles, and she specializes in elder issues. She resides in Jasper. Mary Care, RN, was reelected to the board three years ago. She is the executive director of Valley Hospice and has served nine years on the board. Cindy Donnelly has been a member of the board for 19 years. She is a former reporter with the *Middleboro Sentinel* and lives in Mifflenville. Walter Graham was recently elected to fill a board vacancy created by a resignation. His first term has two years remaining. He is the senior administrator at Medical Associates, a multispecialty group practice located in Jasper and Middleboro. Matty O'Brien, OT, has been a member of the board for seven years. She is professor emeritus of occupational therapy at State University and has lived in Middleboro for the past ten years.

Board Committees, 2014	Chair	Members
Executive	Myer	Ruseski, Steel, Meadows
Finance	Bond	Blau, Logic, Giles, Martin
Professional Advisory	Vosper	Metz, Doe, Care, O'Brien, Ellis
Publicity and Public Relations	Fisher	Donnelly, Black
Building and Grounds	Shields	Graham, George

Mark Shields has been a member of the board for 17 years and is the chair of the building and grounds committee. He resides in Statesville, where he operates a large feed and grain business and serves as an elected town official. Conner George has been a member of the board for 13 years, lives in Mifflenville, and has a professional background in landscaping. Dennis Martin lives in Jasper and is a retired superintendent of schools in Jasper. He has been on the board for four years. Frances Black lives in Middleboro, where she is active in civic affairs. She has been on the board for seven years. Jennifer Ellis lives in Jasper, where she maintains a private practice in speech pathology. She has been on the board for two years.

In 2001, the board created a community advisory council to provide advisory services to each of the programs provided by the agency and to increase community participation without expanding the formal board of directors. Because of the increased possibility of conflict of interest in a competitive healthcare market, as well as declining attendance at quarterly meetings, the board abandoned this council in 2011. It should be noted that in 2010, the board passed a resolution that stated, "Board members represent themselves, not their employers."

Physician interest in serving on the board has been nonexistent since Maynard Cushing, MD, completed his service in 2010. Dr. Rita Hottle of Middleboro serves as the agency's medical director. For the past three years, the agency has experienced a decline in operating margin. In 2013 and 2014, the agency experienced its first losses from operations. The losses were funded out of net assets.

The finance committee is concerned by the downward trend in financial performance from operations as well as the impending significant change in reimbursement for the agency, mandated by the changes in Medicare and Medicaid.

MANAGEMENT TEAM

Hired at the time of corporate expansion in 2010, Martha Washington, RN, MHA, is HCHHA's executive director. Prior to serving in this position, Washington was the regional director for a large for-profit chain of home health agencies, and she managed the affairs of 13 separate agencies. Before that, she was director of marketing for a large medical products firm headquartered in Capital City. She also has approximately ten years of experience as a visiting nurse with a large visiting nurses association located in a major midwestern city. Today, she is vice president of the State Home Health Association and maintains an active presence in the state legislature, lobbying for home care issues. After formal review, the board recently extended her four-year contract for another four years with an increase in salary.

Since her arrival, Washington has reorganized the agency into three divisions: Home Care, Private Duty, and Community Health. As approved by the board prior to her appointment, she opened an additional office located in Jasper to support all programs. Under her leadership, existing services were expanded and new services were added. Above all else, she has worked to ensure that the agency continues to fulfill its mission.

Her management style emphasizes the delegation of clearly expressed responsibilities. She has delegated responsibility for operations to each full-time division manager, added a special assistant to the executive director to assist with projects related to human resources administration and marketing, and upgraded the bookkeeper position to a professional position as controller.

In her first year at the agency, Washington—with the able assistance of select board members and consultants—selected and installed an electronic medical record and patient care planning system specifically designed for home health care. The system has been operational for 18 months in the Home Care Division and 12 months in the Private Duty division. The system required a significant financial commitment.

Ruth Martin, RN, is the manager of the Community Health Division. Four years ago she asked the board to relieve her as executive director, a position she had held for three years. She asked to be retained by the agency as the program manager for the Community Health Program, which upon reorganization became the Community Health Division. The board, after much discussion, agreed and then recruited Washington as executive director with the understanding that Martin would be retained for at least three years. Prior to being appointed executive director, Martin had been the assistant director for 12 years. During this tenure she was responsible for beginning the high blood pressure and maternal and child health program initiatives. Prior to relocating to Middleboro, she was employed by the Capital City Home Health Agency as a home care coordinator. She is a graduate of a southern university and has completed her graduate education in community health nursing.

Catherine Newfields, RN, is the manager of the Home Care Division. Washington hired her in 2011. She is a former assistant professor of community health nursing at State University. Prior to her faculty appointment, Ms. Newfields completed her graduate studies in community health nursing at a major southern university and has 17 years of experience in all aspects of home care, including a brief tenure as the executive director of a small visiting nurses association in another part of the state.

Michael Carlstead, LPN, manages the Private Duty Division. He has more than 30 years of experience as a home health aide (HHA) and licensed practical nurse (LPN). He completed his nursing training 18 years ago and recently earned his bachelor's degree in business administration from a small college that offers distance education opportunities for working professionals. Carlstead has been affiliated with the agency for 24 years and plans to retire in six months.

Steve Callahan is the controller. Washington promoted him upon completion of his bachelor's degree in accounting two years ago. He has worked for the agency for ten years. He was originally hired as assistant bookkeeper and then promoted to bookkeeper. He is currently matriculating part-time for his graduate degree in business administration at State University. Since his promotion, he has become very active in the State Home Care Association.

Judy Herman, RN, is the quality improvement and utilization review manager. Herman devotes most of her time to the Home Care Program and regulatory compliance with Medicare and Medicaid. She is also responsible for the electronic medical record system. She is a graduate of State University and holds an MS in nursing quality improvement from a private university. She has approximately 15 years' experience in quality improvement in home care and worked with Ms. Washington prior to coming to this agency.

Washington has indicated that she is not yet satisfied with the agency's ability to qualify for Medicare reimbursement under the Home Health Prospective Payment System. "The coordination between our clinical personnel and our business office needs to be improved. For example, last year we had more than 20 cases where we failed to adhere to the 60-day physician review requirements. Also, too often we need to begin providing home care services before we actually have the signed physician's certificate, thereby jeopardizing and delaying our qualification under Medicare. These remain some of the issues that Steve Callahan and Catherine Newfields need to address. I am, however, delighted that Steve has taken on an active role with our state association. We need someone who is on top of Medicare's Outcome and Assessment Information Set and in a position to represent our interests."

When interviewed, Steve Callahan indicated that the agency is attempting to address some major problems including "our operating margin and days in accounts receivable. We have some specific challenges that are taking a great deal of attention."

Mary Bird is responsible to Martha Washington for special projects involving human resources administration and marketing, and she staffs the Jasper office when needed. She completed her baccalaureate-level studies in health services administration at State University two years ago, then returned to Middleboro, where she was born. During her academic career, she had interned under Washington when Washington was the regional director for the for-profit chain of home care agencies. She has told Washington that unless her position is made full time in 2015, she will be forced to look elsewhere for employment.

Every two weeks the management team meets formally to review operations and to solve problems. The entire management team attends all monthly board meetings. Washington used the opportunity created by her recent performance review to share certain confidences with the board. She indicated that the Jasper plan needed a complete reevaluation and that she was unsure exactly what an office location in Jasper was really gaining for the agency. She also noted that she had learned that Unicare Homeco, a national for-profit home care corporation, had recently completed a feasibility study to enter the Jasper market.

She indicated that more time was needed to meet personally with major referral sources and that additional funds were needed for advertising. She also said that she was not pleased with the overall decline in financial performance of the agency, particularly in the Community Health Division, and that she foresaw a steadily declining revenue picture in that area. She mentioned to the board that her relationship with Martin, while professional, seemed to highlight the difference in their perspectives and the old versus the new approaches she was attempting to implement. She also stated that to continue expanding services, she would need more help and that she felt that the long-term care program offered by the Home Care Division faced an expanding market.

Washington also said that she faced some "productivity problems" with some of the older employees and alerted the board that some changes may need to be made. Repeatedly, the board emphasized to her that it wants the HCHHA to remain the sole provider of Medicare-certified home care services in the county and that it expected the public to so value the agency that they would continue to support the agency with their contributions. William Bond, chair of the finance committee also indicated to her that he and the rest of the board felt comfortable with her at the helm. The board felt that she understood the finances as well as the dynamics of the home care market. Bond was cautiously optimistic about the financial future as long as the long-term care program matured countywide and as long as the agency could operate effectively under the prospective fixed-price reimbursement environment imposed by Medicare. Myer assured her of board support if the Community Health Division had to be resized and refocused to correspond better with its financial support.

Washington expressed her concern over the increased competition in the home care field as well as the changing reimbursement system. In addition to the interest expressed in the Jasper market by a national home care company, she noted that insurance companies and managed care organizations were expressing increasing interest in using home care services. She pointed out the agency's relatively high dependency on government programs, particularly Medicare, in spite of reasonably successful efforts to establish contracts with managed care organizations. A recent article published in the *State Home Care Association Newsletter* reported that the number of agencies consolidating or going out of business altogether had been increasing dramatically within the past six months, primarily as a result of the impact of reimbursement changes.

HOME CARE DIVISION

This program provides nursing (RN and LPN) and other services (e.g., occupational therapy, physical therapy, speech therapy) to patients in their homes. Medicare, Medicaid, and self-pay and private insurance carriers provide funding for this program. Within the past five years, the agency has pursued contracts with local managed care organizations. As a result of these efforts, contracts are in place with Central States Good Health Network and one other commercial HMO. Medicare finances four categories of service: intermittent nursing care; physical, occupational, or speech therapy; medical social services; and intermittent care provided by a home health aide.

RNs assess and monitor all patients. They are responsible for treatment planning, administering medications, and other nursing services. LPNs work as team members in implementing treatment plans and providing assistance with self-care activities within the context of Medicare and Medicaid regulations. Therapists and other contract professionals (e.g., physical therapists, occupational therapists, speech therapists, social workers, nutritionists) are available as consultants and to implement treatment plans.

The division manager is responsible for the development of the treatment plan when a patient enters the active caseload. Case management is then delegated to the appropriate staff member(s). The responsibility for timely patient discharge and case finding rests with the division manager. The division manager is also responsible for the design and implementation of an appropriate quality assurance system. For the past three years, the staff has reported that patients served by this program immediately following a hospital discharge required more intensive services than they had in the past.

This division also provides pediatric services to children who are born prematurely, who are recovering from surgery, or who are experiencing a chronic disease. Special therapy services are also available. Typically, these types of services are covered by medical insurance plans, Medicare, and Medicaid.

When interviewed, Catherine Newfields, division manager, said "staff turnover was a real and—sometimes—a critical issue." Specifically, she indicated that a primary difficulty with this program was her staff's reluctance to provide IV therapy to cancer patients who routinely require 24-hour, seven-day-a-week coverage. She also stated that she was somewhat concerned that hospitals in Capital City were referring their patients living in Jasper to the Capital City Visiting Nurse Association (VNA), not HCHHA, which had been the practice until 2012. She mentioned being annoyed that almost every time she drove into Jasper, she heard a radio commercial extolling the services of the Capital City VNA. She felt an office location in Jasper was needed more for the Community Health Division than for this division since most of "her staff" lived in the Middleboro area and traveled from the Middleboro office of the agency. She also indicated that getting the required physician recertification every 60 days for Medicare patients was a frequent challenge. Medicare's changing definitions and rules (e.g., definition of *homebound*) were also mentioned as a source of stress and frustration.

Newfields has recently obtained the following national data and is considering whether it might be appropriate in special benchmarking studies.

National Utilization Statistics—Home Health

Patients currently being served by home health agency	Rate per 10,000 population
Patients under 65 years of age	16.4
Patients 65 years or older	277.0
Home health care patients discharged past 12 months	
Under 65 years of age	91.0
65 years or older	1,439.3
At time of discharge, patient...	**Percent**
Remained in community	71.5
Transferred to another setting	20.5
Is deceased	2.3
Unknown	5.7

NOTE: *Discharge* means when a case is closed by the home health agency.

Newfields indicated that her division's experience closely parallels the national Medicare percentages by International Classification of Disease Codes (ICDA) and that—similar to the national data—few cases extend over a long time, making the division's mean service time significantly higher than the median values. Current efforts are under way to compare this division's service times with these national statistics.

A recent study done by a student at the state university indicated that on average every Medicare home visit involved an average (round trip) of 11.2 miles. Over the past five years the study showed that one of the hidden costs of services was the price of gasoline.

When asked about her assessment of the agency, Newfields indicated that she had questions about the impact of the three-division model. She indicated that "her Medicare patients" needed stronger nutritional counseling, flu and pneumonia prevention programs, and that formal programs in pain management, fall prevention, and diabetes education needed to be considered but that "these type of programs typically end up in the Community Health Division." As she said, sometimes "our silos get in our way." She stated that her division needed the opportunity to expand its emergency preparedness. She also indicated that Medicare's rule that client eligibility requires a patient to be "homebound" continues to prevent meeting the needs of a number of individuals. "Too often we have to explain to senior citizens that they do not qualify for Medicare Home Care because they are not homebound as defined by Medicare," she said.

PRIVATE DUTY DIVISION

This program began in 2012. Its primary intent is to assist patients with activities of daily living and to provide other services as needed. Medicare does not provide payment for these services. All funds come from Medicaid, self-pay, and private insurance. The division and its programs began for both service and financial reasons. A formal marketing study completed in 2011 indicated a strong demand for these types of services. To date, demand has surpassed expectations. All services are purchased based on an hourly, daily, or weekly charge. Medicaid sets its own hourly rates by service.

PRIVATE DUTY SERVICES

Under this program professional LPNs can be hired to provide assistance with nursing care including medication assistance and blood pressure screenings. RNs provide skilled nursing care under a physician's order, administer medications, and provide other specialized services. As needed physical, occupational, and speech therapy, and social work services are also available.

COMPANION AND HOMEMAKING SERVICES

This service provides trained staff for light housekeeping, grocery shopping, meal preparation, laundry, and similar duties. Homemaker/housekeeper aides provide in-home services.

PERSONAL CARE SERVICES

Clients are provided assistance with bathing and other activities of daily living as well as respite care. Services are provided by personal care attendants.

Overall this program provides a menu of services (and prices) clients can select to meet their needs. No medical authorization is needed. When interviewed, Carlstead stated, "We never seem to have enough staff to meet our clients' needs." He attributes this to the low pay and benefits and says that "not everyone is really suited to provide these types of services." He also stated that the paperwork really "gets me down. Over the past 20 years the paperwork has just increased and increased—it never seems to end." He did say that his loyal staff is great and that he really enjoys working with them and will miss them when he retires.

Clients contract for a specific number of hours per week and are billed at the end of the week. Most clients pay by credit card, although some pay with cash or check. Any client with an outstanding balance for more than two weeks is reviewed and potentially dropped from the programs. For Medicaid to pay, the client must be Medicaid-eligible and the service plan must be approved by Medicaid before services are provided.

Carlstead stated concerns about the human resources dimension of the agency: "It is essential that we have current information of the professional status of all of our employees, but sometimes we don't. Credentialing and background checks are an issue that could get us into trouble." He also indicated that "work rules" need to be the same within each of the divisions and that the current employee handbook was old and out of date, having been published in 2006. "Other issues we face include the poor and potentially unhealthy condition of the client's home sometimes created by a client's inability to care for (too many) family pets," he said.

COMMUNITY HEALTH DIVISION

Unlike in the other divisions of HCHHA, the manager of this division must apply for grants for private, state, and local funds and attend town meetings to secure funding for services.

TELEHEALTH PROGRAM

This program provides home monitoring for individuals with a chronic illness who present a high risk of rehospitalization. It is a cooperative program between the home health agency and both hospitals. Hospitals and attending physicians identify potential patients who are then offered this service free of charge. An HCHHA nurse works with each patient to help him develop self-care skills.

MATERNAL AND CHILD HEALTH PROGRAM

The Maternal and Child Health Program provides educational, direct services, and health screening programs to expectant mothers and their children who are less than one year of age as well as child home care visits for qualifying children up to one year after birth. As-needed bilirubin photo light therapy services are also available. Funding is provided by the state through an annual grant and from Medicaid. All recipients of state public assistance are eligible (without charge) for this service. Others may receive service for a modest contribution. Classes and clinics are also held in Middleboro and Jasper based on funding received from state, county, and town grants. The agency's prenatal program includes a home visit from a maternity nurse to evaluate the health of both the mother and the child, and to provide counseling on breast-feeding, diet, and infant care. This program has been very well received in the community.

HIGH BLOOD PRESSURE SCREENING PROGRAM

This program provides screening for high blood pressure and makes referrals to physicians as required. Screenings are done in public locations, such as shopping centers, churches, and schools throughout the area. Funding for this program is from the United Appeal and is based on an annual application for continued funding. Recently, the United Appeal has requested a comprehensive assessment of the cost effectiveness of this program as a condition of continued funding.

COMMUNITY HEALTH ACTIVITIES PROGRAM

The Community Health Activities Program provides physicals, immunizations, drug and alcohol testing, smoking cessation programs, and health education services, as needed, to high-risk individuals. All services provided under this program are done at the agency's offices in Middleboro and Jasper. Physicals and immunizations required for public elementary and secondary schools are provided free of charge to any resident of the area. Special classes are held in several areas, including nutrition, foot care, and for stroke patients and their families. Financial support for this program comes from annual appropriations from each town. These appropriations are voted on annually in each town.

SENIOR HEALTH CLINICS

These clinics provide services that include foot care, blood pressure monitoring, earwax removal, injections, medication management support, immunization, and other basic preventive services. Senior health clinics are offered free to all seniors over age 65; younger seniors can pay a modest fee. Clinics are held monthly in Jasper and Middleboro and approximately once every two months in other towns in the country. Support for this program is provided by a grant from the state.

HEAD LICE PROGRAM

Services are provided based on referrals from school nurses. Services include education, prevention, and treatment. Services are available at both offices by appointment. The program is totally financed by an annual grant from the Retail Pharmacy Association of Hillsboro County.

OTHER PROGRAMS

This division also manages the agency's speakers bureau and provides formal classes in first aid and CPR.

When interviewed, Martin stated that she was concerned that more needs were being left unfulfilled because of the lack of funds. She indicated that state and town funding appeared adequate but that she might have a problem in the future "making ends meet." She did say, however, that the United Appeal has expressed concern that the agency had been "so active and successful in its own fund raising, that future allocation decisions [funding to the agency from the United Appeal] would be weighed carefully against the more substantial needs of other worthy organizations."

Issues related to the agency's need for continued outside or community funding were highlighted in a recent letter to the editor of the local paper, in which a family member of an agency client expressed her anger at having to pay for services delivered "by an agency that is supposed to be there for the community, which turns a large profit every year, and which we support through the United Appeal."

Martin expressed concern that the agency was attempting to meet the "needs" of the middle class and becoming less oriented to the "real health needs in the area." She did indicate that a need for adult day care and respite care existed in the community. When asked about the operation of her division, she indicated that she has a positive relationship with her staff, people she has worked with for many years, but that she was concerned that the board and management "seemed to favor the other divisions." She also stated that her division's relationship with the Hillsboro County Health Department was mixed. "We probably need to meet more often, and they typically want us to take on contracts for less than our costs. We have issues with them."

FINANCIAL ISSUES

Medicare and Medicaid cover the services provided by the Home Care Division. Both pay the agency on a prospective basis, with no retrospective settlement. For Medicare, the prospective payment is based on the scoring attributed to the acuity level of the patient at a rate determined by federal guidelines. In 2011 the national standardized payment rate from Medicare was $2,1989.58 per 60-day service period. This rate was 18 percent higher than the rate received by the HCHHA. The most recent national data for home health services indicates that the average payment (all sources) per visit was $145.99. On average a home care agency receives approximately $5,216 per patient served. For Medicaid, the prospective payment is based on a statewide rate per service. When services are rendered to individuals not covered by Medicare or Medicaid, bills are issued either directly to the patient or to the patient's insurance carrier.

The Private Duty Division issues a bill for all services rendered. Every service has a specific hourly charge. Expenses associated with travel to and from the client's home are built into these rates. Medicare does not cover any service provided by this division. Medicaid covers select services that must be preapproved and has a fee schedule for specific services. Most of the revenue earned in this division is from self-pay and commercial insurance.

The Community Health Division finances its services through grants from the state or local agencies. Some towns also provide support as a line item in their budgets. Modest user fees are solicited when appropriate.

Each division is managed as a distinct financial entity and is allocated a portion of the overall agency's general and administrative costs. Managers prepare budgets approximately six months prior to implementation. The board's finance committee reviews Washington's recommended budget; the entire board approves it. The finance committee also oversees budget implementation and examines all significant budget variances.

OTHER INFORMATION

The overall reputation of HCHHA is positive. The agency is known for its prudent administration of funds, high quality of care, and can-do attitude. It is considered by area health professionals to be a highly professional place to work.

The Middleboro office is located in the Hartsdale House, a spacious home on the border of Middleboro's central business district. This house is noted for its antiques. Ample parking is available as this historic home is located on approximately 11 acres. Hartsdale House is a community landmark and is featured in area travel brochures. The Hartsdale family donated this location to the agency in 1979 with a restricted endowment to ensure its physical upkeep and maintenance in perpetuity. The current market value of the property is approximately $1,200,000. The agency is slowly retiring a multiyear loan to modernize the building and install fire warning and sprinkler systems. A motion at a recent board meeting to consider selling this house and use the proceeds for the endowment was defeated. The Jasper office is located in rented space in a professional office building in downtown Jasper.

Twelve years ago the agency received a restricted $960,000 bequest from a former patient "to ensure that quality home care services can be provided to all residents of the area regardless of their ability to pay." The annual fundraising Holiday Ball at the Middleboro Country Club remains a highlight on the local social calendar; additional fund raising events each year include an antique auction, a spring fashion show, a walkathon, and a holiday ornament sale. All philanthropic events are arranged by a local volunteer, Nora Fisher (whose husband serves on HCHHA's board), and her many friends.

On the negative side, a letter recently appeared in the local newspaper asking why a Medicare-certified hospice was not available within the county. The letter suggested that Medicare patients were being denied a valuable benefit because the local health agencies could not "get their acts together." Four years ago this agency decided not to merge with the local hospice, in order to provide these services. When recently asked by a news reporter for a response, both Myer and Washington indicated that the board would reconsider the idea of a Medicare-certified hospice during the next few months.

Last year, news articles in the *Middleboro Sentinel* and on TV Channel 32 on care for the terminally ill highlighted a study released by the state medical society. The medical society's study indicated "approximately 61 percent of all hospice patients have primary diagnoses of neoplasms, with cancer of the lungs, colon, and prostate accounting for 50 percent of all neoplasms." The report continued, "The second-largest group was congestive heart failure, accounting for 45 percent of the admitting diagnosis for this group." On the interview conducted on TV Channel 32, city council members Jennifer Kip and Alan Simpson referred to the lack of a Medicare-certified hospice as "still another indicator as to why new blood is needed in Middleboro—the residents of Middleboro should not be denied this service merely because its home health agency is too busy serving clients from other towns." As a result of this report and the board's concern, the HCHHA engaged consultants to estimate the need for a Medicare-certified hospice in Hillsboro County. The following was extracted from the consultant's reports:

Medicare-Certified Hospice Planning Parameters

National studies indicate that approximately 55 percent of all individuals who die from cancer enroll in hospice services prior to their death. Noncancer enrollees include individuals who died from heart disease (12 percent); dementia, including Alzheimer's disease (11 percent); lung disease (8 percent); stroke (4 percent); kidney disease (3 percent); liver disease (2 percent); HIV/AIDS (0.6 percent); and all other causes (11 percent).

On average enrollees in a Medicare-certified hospice are enrolled for approximately 68.5 days prior to death. Note that 31 percent of enrollees died or were discharged from hospice in seven days or less. Studies also indicate that most hospice care is regular care provided in a patient's home based on periodic visits and home visits as needed.

Nationally, Medicare-certified patient care days are classified as routine care (96 percent), continuous (24-hour) home care (1 percent), inpatient respite care (1 percent), and hospital general inpatient care (2 percent). These same studies indicate that approximately 85 percent of all patients of a Medicare-certified hospice are covered by Medicare, 4 percent are covered by private insurance, and 6 percent are covered by Medicaid. Currently the maximum rate paid by Medicare is $150 per day of routine care, $850 per day for continuous home care, $160 per day for inpatient respite care and $650 per day for general inpatient care. Also, the total annual cost per case cannot exceed $23,000 per hospice enrollee.

Recently, Myer received a letter from a former patient. The letter indicated that the patient had been a long-term contributor to the agency and was very displeased to learn that she would have to pay so much to secure the services of a nurse after her Medicare eligibility ran out. Myer promised to bring this concern to the board.

Both hospitals continue to contract with a private duty nurse, Amy Edwards, RN, and her associates for in-home IV therapy. Edwards also accepts referrals from out-of-area hospitals. It should be noted that on three occasions she has rejected an offer of employment from the HCHHA. She prefers to work independently and bill her services privately or through the hospital. Washington recently learned from a former colleague that Edwards has been in contact with a regional chain of for-profit home health agencies and requested information about establishing a franchise in Middleboro. Edwards has also been contacted by the administrator of Rock Creek, a private, long-term care facility in Mifflenville, and asked to provide them a feasibility study for establishing a private home care agency to serve the greater Middleboro area. Edwards's husband, Keith, is mayor of Middleboro.

Board member David Ruseski recently returned from a statewide conference on home health and has asked for a management assessment of the staff's productivity. At this meeting he learned that national standards exist that could be applied to the agency's acute care program and home health program. For example, Ruseski indicated that a recent national study presented at this meeting used 1.35 hours of nurse time as the average time for an initial home visit and 1.1 hours as the standard time for a continuing care visit done by either an RN or LPN. Note that Washington has recently reported to the board that approximately 20 percent of all home visits done by the Home Care Division are initial visits and that (on average) travel time to and from a home from the Middleboro office is 20 minutes, with a standard deviation of 18 minutes. Currently, all staff assigned to the Home Care Division work out of the Middleboro office.

Last month Washington sent to the executive committee, including Mr. Ruseski, the following national productivity standards she plans to use to assess staff productivity.

Home Health Visit Staff Productivity Profiles (National Standards, 2013)

Staff	Visits per 8-hour shift
RN	4.90
LPN	5.90
HC aide	5.17
Physical therapist	5.39
Occupational therapist	5.25
Social worker	3.20

NOTE: Does not include travel time.

William Bond, chairman of the board's finance committee, has expressed considerable interest in evaluating the likely impact of continuing changes in the Medicare reimbursement system. At a recent board meeting he expressed concern as to whether the agency could continue to stay unaffiliated with at least one of the area hospitals.

When the staff nurses were interviewed most indicated that "doing the required paperwork from home after work was a burden and responsibility that should be recognized and compensated." Some remember the "good old days" when they began and ended their workday at the office. "Today, we rarely go to the office in the morning, we go directly to the client's home and sometimes—but not always—stop at the office in the middle or end of the day. We do the progress notes and other required paperwork from our laptops."

Additional information regarding HCHHA staffing, utilization, fee structure, referral sources, financial status, patient demographics, and quality measures may be found in the following tables.

Position	2014 Salary	2014 FTE	2013 Salary	2013 FTE	2012 Salary	2012 FTE
Administration						
Executive director	125,040	1.0	120,500	1.0	120,500	1.0
Medical director	50,000	0.1	50,000	0.1	50,000	0.1
Special assistant	34,000	0.5	30,000	0.5	30,000	0.5
Controller	61,500	1.0	58,500	1.0	56,500	1.0
Bookkeeper	32,000	2.0	30,670	2.0	30,100	2.0
Secretary	23,950	1.0	22,950	1.0	22,020	1.0
Receptionist, Middleboro	24,000	1.0	22,000	1.0	20,000	1.0
Receptionist, Jasper	26,300	0.5	25,330	0.5	24,303	0.5
Home Care Division						
Manager	74,187	1.0	71,500	1.0	67,000	1.0
RN	53,330	35.5	52,000	35.5	51,000	32.5
LPN	37,376	6.0	36,294	6.0	35,494	8.0
Home health aide	22,900	7.5	22,000	8.0	21,560	8.0
Physical therapist	71,700	3.0	71,000	3.0	70,500	2.2
Occupational therapist	64,480	1.0	64,000	1.0	62,340	0.8
Speech therapist	63,253	0.5	60,338	0.5	61,230	0.5
Secretary	24,300	0.5	21,000	1.0	20,075	1.0
Social worker	43,200	1.0	44,325	1.0	44,000	1.0
Private Duty Division						
Manager	73,000	1.0	71,500	1.0	65,000	1.0
RN	53,330	1.0	52,000	1.0	58,500	1.0
LPN	37,376	7.0	36,294	6.0	27,500	4.0
Personal care attendants	19,451	10.0	19,100	8.0	20,453	4.0

TABLE 2.1
Agency Staffing in FTE and FT Salary: December 31, 2012-2014 ($)

TABLE 2.1
Agency Staffing in
FTE and FT Salary:
December 31,
2012–2014

Position	2014		2013		2012	
	Salary	FTE	Salary	FTE	Salary	FTE
Homemaker/ housekeeper aide	22,900	10.0	21,500	8.0	20,433	6.0
Other	71,700	0.1	71,000	0.1	70,500	0.1
Secretary	24,200	1.0	20,440	1.0	19,000	0.5
Community Health Division						
Manager	63,500	1.0	63,500	1.0	63,500	1.0
RN	53,330	3.0	52,000	3.0	43,500	4.0
Secretary	21,670	1.0	21,000	1.0	19,500	1.0
Total FTE		98.2		94.2		84.7

NOTE: Full-time equivalent (FTE) positions are paid for 2,080 hours per year. All full-time employees receive two weeks paid vacation and 13 paid holidays and work 1,896 hours per year. All salaries are expressed as the average salary for that position. Benefit costs are in addition to salary costs.

TABLE 2.2
Service Area Utilization by Town for Calendar Year Ending December 31, 2014

Division	Service	Boalsburg	Carterville	Harris City	Jasper	Middleboro	Mifflenville	Minortown	Stateville	Total
Home Care										
	RN visits	1,702	2,004	3,404	3,220	16,071	3,794	3,020	820	34,035
	LPN visits	330	356	676	666	3,264	725	445	200	6,662
	HHA visits	422	82	823	863	4,904	967	106	263	8,430
	PT visits	150	26	301	605	1,547	335	18	92	3,074
	OT visits	56	59	107	101	490	100	71	30	1,014
	ST visits	10	13	18	20	91	21	11	5	189
	Social worker visits	26	24	47	51	230	53	38	18	487
Private Duty										
	RN in-home hours	73	54	154	194	798	150	61	50	1,534
	LPN in-home hours	794	290	1,241	1,448	7,109	1,571	293	419	13,165
	PCA in-home hours	957	1,487	1,835	1,741	9,479	2,155	1,315	376	19,345
	HHA in-home hours	844	1,513	1,517	1,291	7,658	2,040	1,729	426	17,018
	Other in-home hours	10	43	21	6	64	0	39	8	191
Community Health										
	Ante/postpartum visits	18	38	56	34	190	101	16	23	476
	Child health visits	7	23	11	44	198	131	12	30	456
Senior Health Clinic Attendees by HCHHA Office Location										
	Seen at Middleboro office	15	12	72	0	653	114	12	45	923
	Seen at Jasper office	0	0	0	246	0	0	0	8	254

(This table can also be found online at ache.org/books/Middleboro.)

Division/Program	2014	2013	2012	2011	2010
Home Care					
Unduplicated client census	1,596	1,582	1,578	1,498	1,499
RN home visits	34,035	35,463	35,867	36,304	37,192
LPN home visits	6,662	5,678	5,980	4,823	4,725
HHA visits	8,430	8,230	8,356	8,856	8,923
PT visits	3,074	2,647	2,630	2,240	2,430
OT visits	1,014	993	897	899	903
ST visits	189	165	174	178	156
SW visits	487	472	434	445	342
Total visits	53,891	53,648	54,338	53,745	54,671
Private Duty					
Unduplicated client census	260	225	145		
RN in-home hours	1,534	1,267	1,050		
LPN in-home hours	13,165	12,564	9,160		
Personal care attendant in-home hours	19,345	16,745	14,290		
HHA in-home hours	17,018	11,788	8,304		
Other in-home hours	212	180	210		
Total hours	51,274	42,544	33,014		
Community Health					
Ante/postpartum visits	476	512	500	499	412
Child health visits	456	502	656	450	496
Prenatal class enrollees	139	140	123	130	112
Children seen, Middleboro	901	740	634	812	845
Children seen, Jasper	301	222	305	317	328

(continued)

TABLE 2.3
Services to
Patients:
2010–2014
(continued)

Division/Program	2014	2013	2012	2011	2010
High Blood Pressure Program					
People screened	7,456	6,867	7,234	7,124	6,838
MD referrals	398	423	307	456	512
Senior Health Clinics					
Clients seen, Middleboro	923	902	920	934	978
Clients seen, Jasper	254	243	289	389	412

(This table can also be found online at ache.org/books/Middleboro.)

TABLE 2.4
Fee Structure as
of December 31,
2014 ($)

Home Care Division per visit exclusive of discounts and contractual allowances[1]	
RN	95.78
LPN	55.50
HHA	50.00
Physical therapist	80.40
Occupational therapist	74.23
Speech therapist	70.60
Social worker	70.89

Private Duty Division per hour exclusive of discounts[2]	
RN	75.00
LPN	51.00
HHA	33.00
Personal care attendant	35.00
Physical therapist	71.00
Occupational therapist	71.00
Speech therapist	71.00
Social worker	71.00

Other	Immunizations, each	10.00
	Physical examinations	50.00

NOTES: 1. Excludes the cost of travel. Client is billed $0.55 per mile to and from Middleboro office. Medical supplies are billed at cost plus 10%. Medicare Home Care prospective rate is determined by fiscal intermediary based on patient information and diagnosis.
2. Includes the cost of travel to and from Middleboro office. Medical supplies and equipment are billed at cost plus 10%. Medicaid has specific fee schedule. Some managed care and commercial insurance plans must not exceed reimbursement rates.

	2014	2013	2012
Home Care Division			
Self-referral	4.0	2.0	2.0
Family or friend	2.0	3.0	2.0
Physician	34.0	32.0	39.0
Hospital—Webster	13.0	15.0	14.0
Hospital—Middleboro	42.0	40.0	39.0
Hospital—Other	1.0	2.0	0.0
Nursing home	2.0	4.0	2.0
Other	2.0	2.0	2.0
Private Duty Division			
Self-referral	42.0	40.0	42.0
Family or friend	21.0	21.0	20.0
Physician	12.0	15.0	12.0
Hospital—Webster	4.0	3.0	2.0
Hospital—Middleboro	9.0	9.0	12.0
Hospital—Other	0.0	2.0	2.0
Nursing home	7.0	6.0	8.0
Other	5.0	4.0	2.0
	100.0	100.0	100.0

NOTE: Numbers are percentages of all new cases.

	2014	2013	2012
Home Care Division	**6,736,375**	**6,322,329**	**5,936,445**
Less allowances for bad debt	(85,240)	(88,340)	(72,450)
Less contractual allowances	(2,049,283)	(1,737,912)	(1,365,999)
Net revenue	**4,601,852**	**4,496,077**	**4,497,996**
Private Duty Division	**3,165,221**	**2,843,959**	**1,893,345**
Less allowances for bad debt	(65,340)	(45,230)	(24,550)
Less contractual allowances	(18,469)	(12,669)	(8,738)
Net revenue	**3,081,412**	**2,786,060**	**1,860,057**
Community Health Division			
Support from state and towns	208,750	240,000	240,000
United Appeal	20,000	20,000	60,000
Other	1,935	1,257	1,458
Net revenue	**230,685**	**261,257**	**301,458**
Total net operational revenue	**7,913,949**	**7,543,394**	**6,659,511**
Expenses			
Divisional			
Salaries and wages	4,186,227	4,086,160	3,604,595
Fringe benefits	1,255,868	1,022,548	1,021,445
Travel	725,388	701,383	604,387
Supplies	453,778	398,202	258,304
Equipment	152,430	122,494	82,394
Total divisional	6,773,691	6,330,787	5,571,125
Administrative			
Salaries and wages	360,233	340,229	335,110
Fringe benefits	102,339	98,334	96,990
Supplies	157,910	158,705	140,680
Equipment	45,929	42,393	34,220

TABLE 2.6

Statement of Revenue and Expenses for Calendar Year Ending December 31 ($)

(continued)

TABLE 2.6

Statement of
Revenue and
Expenses for
Calendar
Year Ending
December 31.
(continued)

	2014	2013	2012
Insurance	56,729	54,202	45,043
Interest	54,894	53,890	53,004
Maintenance—Middleboro	138,595	79,303	78,380
Rent—Jasper office	40,500	40,500	40,500
Computer services	84,253	80,150	73,229
Travel	18,356	18,430	13,450
Heat/light—Middleboro	11,488	10,004	7,545
Legal/audit	55,088	44,411	28,340
Printing and postage	15,540	13,450	12,000
Telecommunications	21,364	19,560	18,334
Staff development	10,060	7,010	7,500
Board expenses	10,150	10,445	6,342
Publications and memberships	10,700	10,500	8,550
Depreciation expense	38,240	39,440	44,350
Total administrative	**1,232,368**	**1,120,956**	**1,043,567**
Total expenses	**8,006,059**	**7,451,743**	**6,614,692**
Gain (or loss) from operations	92,110	91,651	44,819
Other Income	202,445	245,300	295,606
Gain (or loss)	110,335	336,951	340,425

(This table can also be found online at ache.org/books/Middleboro.)

	2014	2013	2012
Current assets			
Cash	708,339	474,519	378,495
Accounts receivable (net)	1,430,404	1,152,383	904,871
Prepaid insurance	8,650	17,340	14,230
Inventory	19,299	19,345	14,236
Total current assets	**2,166,692**	**1,663,587**	**1,311,832**
Property and equipment			
Gross, property & equipment	2,328,440	2,255,606	2,153,284
(Less acccumulated depreciation)	(603,559)	(565,319)	(525,879)
Net property and equipment	**1,724,881**	**1,690,287**	**1,627,405**
Other assets			
Investments (at market)	7,951,190	8,403,134	7,456,012
Total assets	**11,842,763**	**11,757,008**	**10,395,249**
Liabilities and net assets			
Current liabilities			
Accounts payable	487,220	433,291	415,073
Accrued items	284,570	255,683	306,492
Current portion of long-term debt	68,244	69,262	70,385
Total current liabilities	**840,034**	**758,236**	**791,950**
Noncurrent liabilities			
Loan payable	448,292	472,445	492,558
Total liabilities	**1,288,326**	**1,230,681**	**1,284,508**
Net assets			
Donor-restricted fund	6,917,307	6,961,213	5,423,731
Investment fund (at market)	3,024,604	3,062,923	3,521,770
Working capital fund	612,526	502,191	165,240
Total net assets	**10,554,437**	**10,526,327**	**9,110,741**
Liabilities + net assets	**11,842,763**	**11,757,008**	**10,395,249**

TABLE 2.7

Balance Sheet as of December 31 ($)

(This table can also be found online at ache.org/books/Middleboro.)

Percent of AR by Average Days as Receivables, Three-Year Average					Percent of 2014 Total Net Revenue (%)
Average Days in AR by Payer	**30 or Fewer Days**	**31–60 Days**	**61–120 days**	**More Than 120 Days**	
Home Care Division					
Medicare	25	28	38	9	72.5
Medicaid	10	45	40	5	13.5
Commercial insurance	60	25	10	5	10.7
Managed care	45	45	9	1	1.4
Self-pay	78	15	5	2	1.9
Private Duty Division					
Medicare	0	0	0	0	0
Medicaid	5	45	45	5	12
Commercial insurance	35	55	5	5	21
Managed care	25	30	40	5	4
Self-pay	30	60	5	5	63

Community Health Division

The agency bills each grant source, including divisions of government, 1/12 of the total grant amount on the first of a month. On average, 30% is received within 30 days of billing, and 70% is received within 31–60 days of billing. The only exception is the United Appeal grant that is received in total on July 1.

Division	Percent of All Patients			Length of Service (Days)	
	All	Male	Female	Mean	Median
Home Care Division					
Under 65 years	29.50	39.90	23.90	474.00	83.00
Under 18	1.00				
18–44 years	9.20				
45–64 years	19.30				
65 years or older	70.50	60.10	76.10	242.00	64.00
65–69 years	7.10				
70–74 years	10.20				
75–79 years	16.80				
80–84 years	14.50				
85 years or older	21.90			270.00	91.00
Private Duty Division					
Under 65 years	34.50	12.10	35.70	48.50	54.60
18–44 years	5.60				
45–64 years	28.90				
65 years or older	65.50	87.90	64.30	63.70	68.20
65–69 years	14.30				
70–74 years	18.20				
75–79 years	19.30				
80–84 years	5.30				
85 years or older	8.40				

TABLE 2.9
Characteristics of HCHHA Discharged Patients for the Three-Year Period ending December 31, 2014

TABLE 2.10
HCHHA Quality Scorecard: Most Recent Data

	HCHHA	State Average	National Average
Managing daily activities			
How often patients got better at walking or moving around	58%	54%	58%
How often patients got better at getting in and out of bed	54%	48%	54%
How often patients got better at bathing	62%	68%	66%
Managing pain and treating symptoms			
How often the home health team checked patient for pain	96%	96%	98%
How often the home health team treated patient's pain	94%	98%	98%
How often patient has less pain when moving around	62%	62%	67%
How often the home health team treated heart failure (weakening of the heart) patient's symptoms.	92%	99%	98%
How often patient's breathing improved	54%	60%	63%
Treating wounds and preventing pressure sores (bed sores)			
How often patient's wounds improved or healed after an operation	91%	86%	89%
How often the home health team checked patient for the risk of developing pressure sores	100%	96%	98%
How often the home health team included treatments to prevent pressure sores in the plan of care	100%	88%	96%
How often home health team took doctor-ordered action to prevent sores	92%	93%	95%
Preventing harm			
How often the home health team began its patient's care in a timely manner	92%	92%	91%
How often the home health team taught patients (or their family caregivers) about their drugs	87%	86%	91%

(continued)

	HCHHA	State Average	National Average
How often patients got better at taking their drugs correctly by mouth	47%	46%	48%
How often the home heath team checked patient's risk of falling	98%	91%	95%
How often the home heath team checked patients for depression	99%	97%	97%
How often the home heath team determined whether patients received a flu shot for the current flu season	62%	78%	68%
How often the home health team determined whether its patients received a pneumococcal vaccine	68%	69%	66%
For patients with diabetes, how often the home health team got doctor's orders, gave foot care, and taught patients about foot care	96%	92%	92%
Preventing unplanned hospital care			
How often home health care patients needed any urgent, unplanned care in the hospital emergency room without being admitted to the hospital	13%	15%	11%
How often home health care patients had to be admitted to the hospital	28%	25%	26%
Patient survey results			
How often the home health team gave care in a professional way	88%	89%	88%
How well the home health team communicated with patients	87%	88%	85%
How often the home health team discussed medicines, pain, and home safety with patients	83%	85%	83%
How patients rated the overall care from the home health agency	82%	87%	84%
How often patients would recommend the home health agency to friends and family	79%	80%	79%

TABLE 2.10
HCHHA Quality Scorecard: Most Recent Data (continued)

TABLE 2.11
Medicare Home
Health Utilization
by Most Common
Diagnoses: 2014
Data

	ICD Code	Percent of All Patients (National Data)	National Mean Length of Service (Days)	National Median Length of Service (Days)	Percent of HCHHA Patients
Diseases of the circulatory system	390-459	12.6	412	93	15.3
Endocrine, nutritional, and metabolic diseases and immunity disorders	240-279	11.7	410	89	11.2
Diseases of the musculoskeletal system and tissue	710-739	12.6	365	79	14.4
Diseases of the respiratory system	460-519	8.6	308	73	7.3
Diseases of the skin and SC tissue	680-709	6.2	189	73	6.2
Diseases of the nervous system	320-389	4.8	612	327	4.9
Neoplasms	140-239	3.5	138	48	4.3
Diseases of the genitourinary system	580-629	2.6	232	79	3.0
Diseases of the digestive system	520-579	2.3	261	44	2.1
Cumulative total		64.9			68.7

,

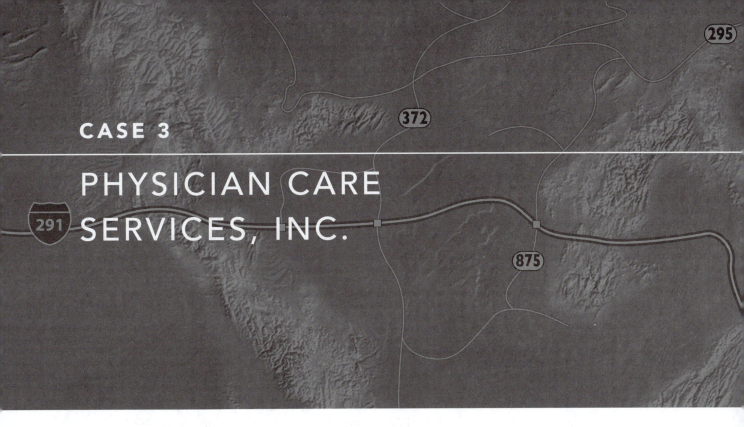

CASE 3

PHYSICIAN CARE SERVICES, INC.

Physician Care Services, Inc. (PCS), was founded as a for-profit corporation on January 1, 2000. Three physicians each own 20 percent of the stock, and one physician owns 40 percent. PCS currently offers nonemergent care services in two locations—at the Alpha Center just outside the city limits of Middleboro in Mifflenville and at the Beta Center in Jasper, close to the Jasper industrial park and suburban neighborhoods. At these locations ambulatory medical care is provided on a walk-in basis. PCS centers do not offer emergency services. If a patient arrives needing emergency services, an ambulance is called to transport the patient to the nearest hospital emergency department.

The Alpha Center opened in January 2000. Originally, it only treated occupational health clients. This policy was changed in 2004 when private patients were accepted. The Beta Center opened in January 2006 and has always treated private as well as occupational health clients.

PCS specializes in providing services that are deemed convenient by the general public. Patient satisfaction remains its highest operational goal. At present, staff physicians employed by PCS do not provide continuing medical care. PCS physicians refer patients to area physicians as warranted for continuing and/or specialized medical care. Although patients often return to a PCS center, chronic illness management is not provided.

PATIENT SERVICES

OCCUPATIONAL HEALTH CLIENTS

Occupational health clients are sent to a PCS center by their employer for treatment of a work-related injury (which is usually covered by workers' compensation insurance), for pre-employment or annual physicals, and for health testing, which are paid for directly by the employer. Because of special work conditions, usually involving hazardous chemicals or materials, some local corporations contract with PCS to provide comprehensive physicals in accordance with Department of Transportation and other federal and state laws and regulations. Local corporations consider PCS a cost-effective and convenient alternative to a hospital emergency department. These corporations use PCS in lieu of employing a physician. Corporate clients expect PCS to assist with all phases of case management involving worker injury. They hold PCS accountable that their workers receive timely, appropriate, and cost-effective services.

Physicals for Occupational Safety and Health Administration compliance are currently priced between $300 and $500 each. Physicals for local police and fire include pulmonary function tests (PFT), laboratory tests, and electrocardiograms (EKGs). They are currently priced between $250 and $350 per physical, depending on contractual volume. Pre-employment physicals are typically priced between $60 and $95 and include a urine dip test. Services provided for occupational health clients are billed directly to the employer.

PRIVATE (RETAIL) CLIENTS

Private clients also seek medical care from PCS centers. All aspects of general medical care are provided except OB/GYN. Private patients are attracted to PCS because they do not need an appointment. PCS accepts cash, checks, and credit cards at time of service. As of 2008, PCS directly bills the larger health insurance plans covering its market area:

- ◆ Statewide Blue Shield

- ◆ American Health Plan

- ◆ Cumberland River Health Plan

- ◆ Central State Good Health Plan

At time of service, retail clients covered by these plans are screened to verify eligibility and to determine whether they have satisfied any required deductibles. If deductibles have been met, patients will be required to pay just the copay amount, and a bill is sent electronically to the insurance plan for the account's balance. If deductibles have not been met, then the patient will pay the bill at time of service, and PCS will enter the bill into the insurance company's system as partial fulfillment of any outstanding deductible. If the patient does not have coverage from one of these insurance companies, she receives a bill to claim reimbursement directly from her insurance plan. PCS also directly bills Medicare. A recent study suggested that these four private insurance companies and Medicare cover approximately 85 percent of PCS's private clients.

Any client who has a history of bad debt at PCS or is unable to pay at time of service is referred to a hospital emergency department for service. PCS maintains an aggressive credit and bad debt collection policy and does not serve Medicaid patients.

Patients living within a 30-minute travel distance from a PCS center typically constitute 80 percent of PCS's private pay patients.

ORGANIZATION AND MANAGEMENT

Each center is located in approximately 6,000 square feet of rental space devoted to patient services. The Alpha Center is located on main roads between Middleboro and Mifflenville in a small shopping center. The Beta Center is located on the first floor of a new office building adjacent to a large shopping mall in Jasper. Ample parking is provided in both locations. Each center maintains attractive signs.

Each center is open 60 hours per week, 8:00 a.m. to 7:00 p.m. on weekdays and 9:00 a.m. to 2:00 p.m. on Saturdays. Both centers are closed on Sundays and Memorial Day, July 4, Thanksgiving, Christmas, and New Year's Day. Each center has four fully furnished patient examination rooms and one extra room. Currently each center has some excess space.

For patient care the minimum staffing at each center is one receptionist/billing clerk, one medical assistant, and one physician or nurse practitioner. Additional staff (e.g., advanced registered nurse practitioner, physician assistant, medical assistant) is scheduled based on anticipated high-volume days. Typically the nurse practitioner works on Saturdays and assists with physicals and other services on high-volume days. Physician assistants also assist on high-volume days.

The central administrative and billing office is an additional 2,500 square feet and is located adjacent to Alpha Center. The central office staff includes the president, medical director, director of nursing and patient care, business office manager, and the billing and bookkeeping staff.

CHARGES

Each center uses the same price schedule. The basic visit charge (CPT 99202) has changed each year.

January–December	Private Pay ($)	Occupational ($)
2010	94	161
2011	99	170
2012	104	180
2013	110	189
2014	120	201

Current detailed prices include:

CPT Procedure		
Code	**Description**	**Price ($)**
99201	Office visit, brief, new	96
99202	Office visit, limited, new	120
99203	Office visit, inter, new	201
99204	Office visit, comp, new	226
99211	Office visit, min, est	65
99212	Office visit, brief, est	96
99213	Office visit, limited, est	201
99214	Office visit, inter, est	201
99215	Office visit, comp, est	294

Additional charges are levied for ancillary testing and specialized physician services, such as suturing. A patient returning for a medically ordered follow-up is charged $96 for the return visit. Based on Current Procedural Terminology (CPT) comparison, PCS fee levels are competitive within the area. No similar medical service is offered within a 45-minute radius from each center. In the past—as part of an advertising campaign to attract private pay patients—each May and June PCS has offered discounted physicals, such as camp physicals for children at $48 and for all children in a family for $69.

Steve J. Tobias, MD, board chair and president of PCS, says national studies suggest that urgent care visits are at least $10 less than a visit to primary care physician in private practice. Other studies indicate that urgent care visits cost $250 to $600 less than emergency department visits for the same CPT code.

Some occupational health clients are charged based on a negotiated volume-based price, especially for physicals. PCS's medical director negotiates specific fees for physicals and specific medical tests ordered by an employer. Typically, an employer approaches PCS in need of a specific type of physical, such as the annual physical required by the Department of Transportation for all operators of school buses, or specific medical test for employees. PCS submits a bid to perform a specific number of physicals based on a flat rate per physical.

As of 2007, PCS does its own payroll. Employees must have direct deposit with a local bank. Each employee receives an electronic pay stub biweekly (with accrued balance of vacation and sick time) and a W-2 at the end of the year.

BOARD OF DIRECTORS

The board of directors is composed of the four physician owners and meets quarterly to review operations. The annual board meeting occurs in December, at which time officers are elected for the coming year. As majority stockholder, Dr. Tobias is chairman of the board and president of PCS. Jay T. Smooth, MD, is the board secretary. Other board members are Rita Hottle, MD, and Laura Cytesmath, MD. Current owners have the option of buying any available stock at its current book value. An outsider can purchase stock in this company only if all the current owners refuse to exercise this option and he receives the approval of the existing owners. It should be noted that PCS has paid a stock dividend in three of the last five years.

PRESIDENT AND MEDICAL DIRECTOR

Dr. Tobias is also the medical director of PCS. He is a graduate of the medical school at Private University and has completed postgraduate medical education at Walter Reed Army Hospital in general internal medicine. He is board certified in general internal medicine, emergency medicine, and occupational health. He also holds a master's in public health from State University. As medical director, Dr. Tobias is responsible for medical quality assurance programs and the recruitment and retention of qualified physician employees. He is also responsible for securing the services of consulting radiologists to read all X-rays. He receives a separate salary as medical director and as president. Compensation for the medical director position began in 2008. Before Dr. Tobias founded PCS, he was a full-time emergency physician at Middleboro Community Hospital. He originally worked to establish joint venture urgent care centers with Middleboro Community Hospital. When this approach failed, he recruited the other stockholders and moved ahead with PCS. As president, Dr. Tobias is responsible for the management of all resources and strategic planning.

Dr. Tobias schedules the other physicians and the nurse practitioners. He also works in the centers and provides on-call services as needed. He has consulting medical staff privileges in the Department of Medicine at Middleboro Community Hospital.

CLINICAL STAFF

In total, the clinical staff is composed of seven physicians, three nurse practitioners, and two physician assistants. All physicians hold medical staff privileges at an area hospital.

Name	Medical Specialty	Certification
Bennet Casey, MD	Family practice	Board certified
Mark Welby, MD	Family practice	Board certified
Steve Tobias, MD, MPH **	Emergency medicine	Board certified
Jay Smooth, MD *	Emergency medicine	Board certified
Rita Hottle, MD *	Emergency medicine	Board certified
Laura Cytesmath, MD *	Emergency medicine	Board certified
Micah Foxx, DO, MPH	Occupational health	Board certified
Melisa Majors, MD	Occupational health	Board certified
Carl Withers, ARNP	Family and adult health	
Jane Jones, ARNP	Family and adult health	
Gerri Mattox, ARNP	Family and adult health	
Rutherford Hayes, PA		
Mary Fishborne, PA		

* Owner
** Owner and president

Until 2007, staff physicians were retained as independent contractors and received no benefits above their hourly wage. Beginning in 2007 when nurse practitioners were added, physicians (and all other employees) who worked more than 1,000 hours were provided comprehensive benefits, including family medical coverage. Also as of 2007, PCS reimburses all physicians and nurse practitioners for their medical malpractice insurance. Full coverage is provided when a member of the medical staff works 1,400 hours at PCS. Others receive a partial reimbursement.

Physicians are paid $100 per hour. Nurse practitioners receive $50 per hour. These payment levels have been fixed for two years and are considered within the appropriate market range. Drs. Smooth, Hottle, and Cytesmath also work as emergency physicians at Middleboro Community Hospital. Dr. Casey serves as medical director one day per week at an area corporation, where he specializes in occupational health. Dr. Welby also works at Convenient Med Care, Inc., in Capital City. Dr. Foxx, who recently relocated to Jasper with her family, is available to work no more than six shifts per month, a condition she has established until her children reach school age. Dr. Majors also works as an emergency physician in Capital City. Physician assistants are paid $40 per hour and assist physicians on anticipated high-volume days.

Dr. Tobias schedules all members of the medical staff for work on a monthly basis with the understanding that if a physician is unable to work, it is her responsibility to secure a replacement from the qualified medical staff of PCS. Physicians and nurse practitioners work an entire shift (e.g., 11 hours on a weekday). Fridays and Saturdays are typically assigned to the nurse practitioners. Physician assistants are on call for busy days to assist physicians.

The clinical staff of PCS meets quarterly to review areas of concern. Dr. Tobias does random reviews of medical records to ensure compliance with standards of clinical practice. He is also responsible for all issues involving credentialing.

MEDICAL ASSISTANTS

Medical assistants at each center are trained to take limited X-rays, draw specimens for laboratory testing, do EKGs, and conduct simple vision and audiometric examinations. Each center is equipped to do:

1. On-site X-ray

2. PFT

3. EKG

4. Audiometric and visual testing

5. Some laboratory testing (e.g., strep screen, dip urine)

6. Drug and breath alcohol testing

A regional laboratory processes more advanced laboratory work.

Two medical assistants are assigned to each weekday shift. One is assigned for 7 hours per day (i.e., 35 hours per week) and the other is assigned for 4 hours per weekday and Saturdays (i.e., 25 hours per week). Responsibilities include examination room preparation, assisting the physician or nurse practitioner, patient testing, case management, scheduling visit follow-up care, and addressing patient questions. Each center maintains a pool of qualified medical assistants who are trained, evaluated, and scheduled by the director of nursing and clinical care.

CENTRAL OFFICE STAFF

Dr. Tobias devotes his time to being both the president and medical director at PCS and filling in at a center when needed. As president he is responsible for the overall management of PCS. Joan Carlton, LPN, is director of nursing and clinical care. She trains, supervises, and schedules the medical assistants. She is also responsible for ordering medical supplies, meeting with occupational health employers as needed, and general administrative duties as assigned by Dr. Tobias. If needed, she substitutes for a medical assistant at a center.

Martha Coin directs the business office and has three full-time staff. She schedules the receptionist staff at each center. She and her staff assist the receptionists and billing clerks at each center, manage all insurance billing, and manage the general ledger, including accounts payable and accounts receivable. If needed, she or a member of her staff substitutes for the receptionist at a center. The central office billing staff also maintains a list of available (and trained) fill-in receptionists to cover absences and other needs.

RECEPTIONIST STAFF

One full-time (35 hours per week) front desk receptionist is hired for each center. Aside from greeting and registering all patients, the receptionist is also responsible for appointments, billing, records for occupational clients, and managing cash receipts. One or more additional receptionists are hired for the remaining 25 hours per week.

ADDITIONAL INFORMATION

In 2008 PCS began using URGENT CARE MIS, an electronic medical information, general ledger, and billing system. Computer terminals were installed in the reception area in each center, at the central office, and in each examination room. PCS uses this system for all phases of financial and medical record keeping and billing, appointment services, case management, staff scheduling, and data management. This system captures, stores, and reports all CPT codes and links medical procedures with revenue and expense information. The health insurance billing system has a direct Internet link with the participating insurance companies and Medicare. PCS purchased the hardware and leased the required software for ten years. It receives hardware maintenance, software updates, and technical assistance from the vendor.

A 2013 study of medical records indicated that the most common CPT codes at PCS are

◆ 99212/3 and 99202 Office/Outpatient Visit,

◆ G0001 Drawing Blood,

◆ 85029 Automated Hemogram, and

◆ 71010/2 Chest X-Ray.

Injuries and rechecks generally account for 20 percent of all visits.

Paper medical records that existed prior to 2008 are retained in active file for seven years, and then transferred to closed files.

When interviewed, Dr. Tobias indicated that discharging Nancy Stone, RN, as director of nursing and clinical services in 2012 was a hard decision. Some employees still regret this situation. Stone was well liked but just could not get along with some of the physicians and had a great deal of difficulty coping with multiple job responsibilities. At the end of her tenure she refused to provide patient care as needed at the Beta Center. After she was discharged, Stone complained that she had "too many duties to do well, and PCS was more interested in getting patients in and out than in providing patients quality medical care." She has retained an attorney and informed Dr. Tobias that she is suing him and PCS for "wrongful discharge." As she stated at the initial hearing for the lawsuit, "Meeting job expectations was hard when the job lacked any formal job description." Dr. Tobias shared in the interview that he felt compelled to act even though Stone is the sister of the vice president for human resources at Carlstead Rayon, a growing occupational health client of the Alpha Center, and that additional details are not available given that this case is currently being handled by legal counsel.

Dr. Tobias stated that the owners should look forward to achieving even greater corporate profitability. Dr. Tobias indicated that no one foresaw the terrible first three years of financial losses. He also said that within the past few years, PCS has earned its place in the regional medical care system and its future appears solid. It should be noted that, at the end of 2007, one of the original physician partners, who is no longer affiliated with PCS, exercised his option to be bought out by another stockholder. Dr. Tobias was the only partner willing at that time to increase his ownership in PCS.

Dr. Tobias also indicated that the owners might now be in the position to open a third and even fourth location. He also discussed purchasing buildings to house the existing centers and adding some services to better serve their occupational and private pay clients.

"We are a debt-free corporation that is beginning to earn serious profits," he said. "Along the way we have distinguished ourselves by the high quality of care we have provided—our patients and occupational health clients are delighted with our highest-level commitment to patient care, convenience, and affordable prices. While it has been a long road, I have every reason to believe we will continue to prosper and expand."

The original real estate leases on the Alpha and Beta Centers expire at the end of 2015. Dr. Tobias said that he timed the expiration of these leases to coincide with when PCS would be ready to make a major strategic move. Each current lease has a renewal clause for up to 36 months, with an escalation clause so that rents do not increase more than 15 percent per year. Tobias estimates that appropriate facilities could be acquired for $150 per square foot (including land, site improvements, and facilities) and that it would take approximately six months from the time the contract was executed to when the center could be fully operational.

When asked to identify future challenges, Tobias noted that he felt that volume had just about hit the level at which total service time averages about 20 minutes. He did indicate, however, that there might be a need for larger waiting rooms and that those patients waiting for more than 90 minutes might be a problem. Tobias was, however, pleased that patients generally reported "complete satisfaction" with the quality of care provided by PCS. Dr. Tobias repeatedly cited the competent clinical and administrative staff. Overall, he indicated that he was concerned about continued rapid growth. "Our early success with occupational health may be slowing. If we lose a significant amount of manufacturing in our area, we potentially lose occupational health clients. Our future in occupational health will follow the local economy."

Dr. Tobias noted that regional unemployment has already affected occupation health. Fewer people are being hired and working. Fees paid by the workers' compensation program have been fixed for 24 months. People who are unemployed lack health insurance. Dr. Tobias expressed a great deal of optimism that the full implementation of the new federal health insurance plan (the Patient Protection and Affordable Care Act) would significantly expand PCS's pool of private clients.

Two years ago, PCS instituted an appointment plan for occupational health clients, which Dr. Tobias reported has been very successful. Under this plan, occupational health clients are scheduled for physicals or medical testing. Under the "call before you come" system, patients (or employers) can call ahead to determine the approximate wait time, make a decision, and—if they want service—register for service at an approximate time that day, thereby ensuring themselves a specific place in the queue for service even before they arrive at a center. Every patient who arrives at a center is given an approximate wait time by the receptionist and told they need not wait in the waiting area to preserve the scheduled time for their appointment. While "first in, first out" is generally used, urgent care cases (especially injuries) are bumped ahead of nonemergency patients. Signs in the waiting area explain to patients that some occupational health clients are served by appointment and that appointments override arrival order.

PCS advertises its services in the regional market. It uses billboards on main roads and newspaper advertising. It also uses an extensive website and social media. The director of nursing and patient care visits current and prospective occupational health clients and typically answers approximately 15 to 25 telephone inquiries per month regarding quotes for specific services, such as employee physicals.

When interviewed, other PCS physicians offered different perspectives. Three physicians expressed concern about the manner in which Dr. Tobias schedules the physicians. They were never sure exactly how many shifts per month they would work and at which center. All prefer to work at only one center and indicated that this type of stability leads to a better medical care team.

Records suggest that certain physicians may have productivity profiles significantly different from those of other physicians. It appears that on busy days, revenue per visit drops, a trend that suggests that physicians do less ancillary testing when they are busy. The target for physicians and nurse practitioners is 3 to 4 patients per hour. Three physicians have also requested extra compensation for busy days. They contend that they tend to be scheduled on "very busy days" and receive the same hourly compensation as physicians who work on slower days. Dr. Tobias indicated that he does not feel that their claim is warranted.

In 2010, two (nonowner) physicians said that because they are paid by the hour, they should be paid for the time they spend treating those patients who arrive right before closing time. Up until this change, all staff were only paid for the hours in their shift (e.g., 11 hours), which was sometimes less than the number of actual hours worked. Employees are expected to treat all patients that arrive during working hours even if this extends their work time beyond closing time. All physicians reported that they felt that their pay level was reasonable given their responsibilities.

Six occupational health nurses at area corporations were interviewed. Each indicated that she and her corporation were satisfied with PCS. A number of these nurses indicated that they appreciated PCS—specifically the medical assistants—keeping them informed about specific patients and that PCS was creative in explaining restriction and suggesting "light duty," medically appropriate work an injured worker could perform for the employer as an alternative to her regular duties until she was ready to resume her regular duties.

Dr. Tobias recently returned from a professional meeting with statistics that he felt could help PCS better estimate its future market. These statistics apply to this state:

Average Number of Physician Visits—Ambulatory Care per Person, per Year, by Age and Sex (National Statistics)

Age	Males	Females
0–14	3.37	3.09
15–44	1.99	3.92 (includes OB/GYN)
45–64	2.98	4.34
65+	4.51	5.19

NOTE: Visits unrelated to workers' compensation and occupational health

At this meeting, Dr. Tobias also learned that other urgent care corporations use the following parameters in their fiscal and market planning.

- For every 15 percent increase in a basic visit fee, there will be a 25 percent reduction in utilization of retail patients without health insurance (i.e., who pay by cash, check, or credit card).

- Patients covered by insurance, including Medicare and commercial insurance, are generally not price-sensitive as long as the annual increase in the basic visit fee does not exceed 20 percent.

- Annual increases up to 15 percent in ancillary charges do not affect the number of new visits by retail clients. It appears that ancillary charge increases above 15 percent may reduce return visits by as much as 45 percent regardless of payment source.

At the next board meeting, Dr. Tobias plans to discuss a series of new ideas and opportunities that deserve the board's attention. Currently his ideas and opportunities include the following:

PRESCRIPTION DRUGS FOR RETAIL PATIENTS

This service is currently available to patients covered by workers' compensation. State law allows physicians (and nurse practitioners) to dispense prescription drugs as long as adequate records are maintained. National firms specializing in drug repackaging let PCS buy prepackaged prescription drugs ready for sale to a patient. PCS has already established its formulary for workers' compensation patents. PCS has determined that by maintaining 12 specific drugs in pill form it can meet approximately 60 percent of the retail demand that PCS physicians create for prescription drugs. The charge for prescription drugs for workers' compensation patients is directly billed to the employer as part of the overall charge for service.

Dr. Tobias indicated that PCS should consider extending this service to all patients. By only providing "high-volume" drugs, PCS can guarantee high inventory turnover. An appropriately sized initial inventory for retail patients can be capitalized for a center for $1,000. All suppliers promise a next-day replenishment of inventory items. The shelf life of all drugs is more than one year. Even with a markup of 800 percent, PCS prescription prices will be competitively priced in the area. The question is whether this service should be expanded to retail patients. By reviewing medical records of current retail patients (non-physicals), PCS has determined the number of prescriptions received per visit by patients.

Age of Patients	Average Number of Prescriptions Received per Visit
0–14	1.20
15–44	0.80
45–64	1.10
65+	1.90

The average supplier cost per PCS prescription is estimated to be $5. To maintain the proposed inventory, additional software costing $12,500 per year is required to verify insurance coverage and copays and process insurance payments. Dr. Tobias would like to potentially begin this service within six months. Questions remain, however, whether any prescriptions issued by PCS should be refilled without another medical visit. Questions also remain as to billing procedures when patients do not have a current prescription plan card at time of service. An urgent care center in Capital City recently ended its pharmaceutical sales to retail patients because of the high number of refused claims by drug plans.

DRUG TESTING FOR HEALTHY EMPLOYEES

The director of human resources at a local company, a current PCS occupational health client, has stated that its new labor contract includes a clause stating that "all workers and job applicants are subject to mandatory random drug testing and any worker who fails or refuses the test will be immediately discharged or not hired." The client has asked PCS to perform drug tests on referred workers or job applicants.

Note that under the new state law and workers' compensation regulations, drug testing is also required for all workers who are injured at work. Employers are also able to institute random drug testing. Some other clients have even requested that PCS select some of their workers for testing using a random selection process. A process using employee Social Security numbers has been discussed. Other occupational health clients have previously suggested that PCS begin this type of service.

Currently a test is available from a reference laboratory for a processing cost of $8 per test. Results screen for the presence of all common illegal drugs. The list price for this test is $42 and $63 if a certified medical review officer (MRO) reads the test. Dr. Tobias is a certified MRO. The test requires about 10 minutes of a medical assistant's time, specifically to maintain compliance with the chain of custody protocol during collection.

PHYSICALS BY APPOINTMENT FOR EMPLOYEES

Increasingly, employers are issuing formal requests for proposal (RFPs) for occupational health physicals that require appointments. For example, a current RFP from a local employer is for 350 annual physicals during 2015 that must be done between 3:15 p.m. and 4:30 p.m. Monday through Friday at the Beta Center. (The company's employees work 7:00 a.m. to 3:00 p.m.) The physical must include the following components:

	PCS List Price
Medical history and examination	$70
EKG	$70
X-ray chest	$101
Urine (dip) test	$20
Complete blood count with differential	$40
Vision screen	$27
Audiometric test	$3

Each physical will take approximately 80 minutes to complete. The PCS list price for this package of services and tests is $331. PCS vendor costs for the physical (e.g., X-ray reading fees, laboratory charges) are estimated to be $70.00. The PCS bid for this contract will be evaluated on the basis of total price and fulfilling expectations related to schedule and timing.

Currently, this employer uses the emergency department at Middleboro Community Hospital for all matters involving occupational health. Dr. Tobias feels that the board must develop policies regarding these types of requests.

MANAGEMENT POLICIES CONCERNING WAITING

Dr. Tobias is concerned that patient waiting time may be a problem. *Waiting* appears to be defined by patients as the time they spend in a reception area, not the time they might spend in an examination room waiting to see the clinical staff. National studies indicate that approximately 57 percent of patients coming to an urgent care center wait 15 or fewer minutes.

Dr. Tobias will tell the board that PCS must begin to address this problem after they first have a better understanding of current waiting times and issues. A consultant has told PCS that its service times for retail patients are approximately 20 percent of gross billed charges. For example, a patient visit that costs $100 (gross billed charges) takes approximately 20 minutes—20 percent of 100—of service time. For all workers' compensation cases and employer-paid physicals, service time is approximately 25 percent of gross billed charges.

As demand increases during the day, the clinical care team sequentially sees patients in multiple examination rooms. Typically, a visit begins with a brief encounter with the medical assistant, who records vital signs, takes a medical history, and records the reason for the visit. The physician or nurse practitioner then enters the room (with the chart) and performs an additional examination. Specific medical tests may be ordered. The medical assistant administers these tests (e.g., X-ray) and/or collects blood or urine for laboratory processing. The physician or nurse practitioner ends the visit providing the patient with a specific diagnosis and treatment plan, additional medical orders, or a referral.

AMBULATORY PHYSICAL THERAPY

National studies estimate that approximately 30 percent of the occupational health clients (injuries covered by workers' compensation) and 5 percent of retail clients (nonphysicals) at centers like PCS are referred to physical therapy for treatment. Dr. Tobias has indicated that PCS may have the opportunity to move into this market.

Area providers typically receive $195 from workers' compensation funds for an initial physical therapy evaluation and (on average) $125 per therapy visit. On average each workers' compensation case generates 5.75 visits—an initial visit and 4.75 additional visits. Most commercial and managed care plans pay $60 per visit and $100 for an initial evaluation.

Dr. Tobias has recommended that PCS consider, depending on estimated demand, offering physical therapy services for one or both centers (e.g., 7:00 a.m. to 2:00 p.m. Monday, Wednesday, and Friday and 11:00 a.m. to 7:00 p.m. on Tuesday and Thursday).

Staffing could include one full-time physical therapist (PT) at $80 per hour (or $75,000 plus benefits) and part-time physical therapy assistants (PTAs) at approximately $25 per hour. PTs can simultaneously manage between two and five patients and supervise a PTA, who provides the direct therapy, given specific treatment plans. Dr. Tobias also says that PCS may be able to contract for the needed PT and PTAs from local nursing homes. The PT must do the initial patient evaluation and establish the treatment plan but need not be on site to supervise the PTAs.

Equipment for each center could be purchased and installed for approximately $30,000 (five year depreciation, no salvage value). Operational costs, such as laundry and medical supplies, are estimated to add approximately $15 per visit. The one-time information system upgrade for ambulatory physical therapy would cost $6,500. Other costs may need to be estimated. A consultant has recommended that PCS only service workers' compensation patients to start, but Dr. Tobias indicates that full coverage needs to be considered.

OTHER ISSUES

The board members know that one member of the board will come to the next board meeting in hopes of discussing whether PCS is for sale and how best to position PCS for sale. He believes that PCS cannot be a long-term successful player in the increasingly competitive medical marketplace. He stated, "I am very concerned that the big box stores will add walk-in services to go along with their pharmacies. I just do not see how we can compete. Our market area is just too volatile!" It is known that Dr. Tobias has always said he would be willing to sell PCS for "the right price." He has also stated when the regional economy and manufacturing pick up, PCS's occupational health business should rebound along with its overall profits.

PCS is liable for a 31 percent federal tax and 9 percent state tax on its profits. Carry-forward losses experienced in the initial years of operation have expired. Local real estate taxes on owned land and buildings are 4 percent of assessed valuation. Current assessed valuation of land in the county is approximately 40 percent of market value or total development cost.

Originally three-year renewable leases were used to secure the needed medical equipment (e.g., X-ray machines, computers) and most furniture. In 2005 PCS's accountant recommended that because PCS was now earning a profit and had used all of its carry-forward tax credits, it should consider borrowing funds to purchase needed equipment and should cancel all outstanding equipment leases. Between 2005 and 2007, it did. Each center required between $150,000 and $200,000 worth of new equipment. The only equipment leases that remain are for color copiers and general office equipment. PCS maintains a line of credit with a commercial bank in Capital City. Its cost of capital is 2.5 percent above the *Wall Street Journal* prime rate.

Based on its annual credit review, PCS has been informed that its cost of capital could increase by 1 or 1.5 percentage points over the next 18 months. The bank stated that the management and organization of PCS are seriously flawed: "PCS has become too dependent on Dr. Tobias in his many roles. His duties need to be divided between two or more qualified professionals." If PCS does not address this situation, its credit worthiness will be significantly downgraded. This situation was also noted in the 2013 audit and management letter.

Officials in the City of Jasper have requested a meeting with PCS to discuss emergency planning and expanded services. Their specific questions will include whether PCS would expand hours on Saturday and offer services on Sunday afternoon. Their letter indicated that the majority of urgent care centers nationally offer services on Saturdays (8:00 a.m. to 8:00 p.m.) and Sundays (9:00 a.m. to 7:00 p.m.). A formal response to this inquiry is due within the week.

Additional information regarding PCS utilization, patient demographics, and finances may be found in the following tables.

TABLE 3.1
PCS Utilization Report

	Alpha	Alpha	Beta	Beta	Alpha	Beta	Total
	Total Visits	Private Visits	Occupational Health Visits	Private Visits	Occupational Health Visits	Gross Charges ($)	Gross Charges ($)	Gross Charges ($)
2014								
January	909	302	185	192	230	78,450	94,040	172,490
February	1,030	402	170	207	251	87,650	102,272	189,922
March	1,039	449	165	204	221	92,425	93,092	185,517
April	1,100	481	190	187	242	101,925	96,844	198,769
May	988	480	103	167	238	82,660	92,876	175,536
June	1,067	493	150	195	229	94,625	94,168	188,793
July	1,195	460	252	219	264	112,940	107,748	220,688
August	1,276	503	260	217	296	120,075	116,812	236,887
September	1,031	406	165	209	251	87,050	102,552	189,602
October	1,048	403	233	205	207	101,635	89,144	190,779
November	905	329	225	168	183	90,625	76,956	167,581
December	799	325	230	119	125	91,225	53,160	144,385
Total	**12,387**	**5,033**	**2,328**	**2,289**	**2,737**	**1,141,285**	**1,119,664**	**2,260,949**
2013								
January	894	312	180	202	200	72,228	75,038	147,266
February	990	398	166	214	212	79,732	79,526	159,258
March	1,048	440	173	217	218	86,095	81,413	167,508
April	1,102	486	176	203	237	92,154	84,592	176,746
May	999	476	115	163	245	79,069	81,872	160,941
June	978	478	132	133	235	82,622	75,752	158,374
July	1,031	455	204	117	255	93,925	78,948	172,873
August	1,276	501	251	269	255	108,564	97,036	205,600
September	970	396	160	202	212	78,324	78,098	156,422
October	1,056	447	203	199	207	92,778	76,466	169,244
November	1,005	423	254	178	150	99,867	59,432	159,299
December	1,000	405	240	190	165	94,995	64,685	159,680
Total	**12,349**	**5,217**	**2,254**	**2,287**	**2,591**	**1,060,353**	**932,858**	**1,993,211**
2012								
January	876	303	170	213	190	66,842	73,912	140,754
February	938	365	169	200	204	73,720	75,800	149,520
March	993	402	190	205	196	81,928	74,420	156,348
April	963	406	156	194	207	75,924	75,806	151,730
May	1,001	426	155	175	245	78,014	82,950	160,964
June	986	453	145	143	245	79,192	78,982	158,174

(continued)

	Alpha	Alpha	Beta	Beta	Alpha	Beta	Total
	Total Visits	**Private Visits**	**Occupational Health Visits**	**Private Visits**	**Occupational Health Visits**	**Gross Charges ($)**	**Gross Charges ($)**	**Gross Charges ($)**
July	1,027	451	184	127	265	86,374	81,998	168,372
August	1,259	493	271	227	268	107,692	95,148	202,840
September	909	312	203	189	205	74,138	74,686	148,824
October	1,057	449	213	178	217	91,656	76,322	167,978
November	974	425	207	164	178	87,780	64,836	152,616
December	1,012	401	231	193	187	89,604	70,682	160,286
Total	**11,995**	**4,886**	**2,294**	**2,208**	**2,607**	**992,864**	**925,542**	**1,918,406**
2011								
January	866	313	160	200	193	62,917	60,235	123,152
February	887	375	153	145	214	68,415	58,115	126,530
March	978	397	187	189	205	76,933	61,332	138,265
April	954	376	159	205	214	69,604	64,895	134,499
May	1,035	445	193	165	232	83,245	63,885	147,130
June	1,047	463	193	160	231	85,207	63,125	148,332
July	968	421	195	107	245	80,989	59,866	140,855
August	1,212	504	241	207	260	98,316	74,091	172,407
September	986	323	200	188	275	71,207	74,869	146,076
October	990	409	198	156	227	80,221	61,893	142,114
November	974	400	212	145	217	81,760	58,700	140,460
December	960	394	223	156	187	83,086	54,093	137,179
Total	**11,857**	**4,820**	**2,314**	**2,023**	**2,700**	**941,900**	**755,099**	**1,696,999**

TABLE 3.1
PCS Utilization Report (continued)

(This table can also be found online at ache.org/books/Middleboro.)

Week	Mon	Tues	Wed	Thurs	Fri	Sat	Total
Alpha							
1					20	18	38
2	52	34	27	23	27	26	189
3	53	37	29	24	25	22	190
4	52	33	33	22	21	20	181
5	51	27	24	25	22	16	165
Total	208	131	113	94	115	102	763

TABLE 3.2
Detailed Utilization (Visits—All Types) for August 2014

(continued)

TABLE 3.2
Detailed Utilization
(Visits—All Types)
for August 2014
(continued)

Week	Mon	Tues	Wed	Thurs	Fri	Sat	Total
Beta							
1					19	9	28
2	28	26	14	16	26	12	122
3	28	30	18	14	19	9	118
4	29	25	15	19	21	13	122
5	28	24	18	21	23	9	123
Total	113	105	65	70	108	52	513
Total	321	236	178	164	223	154	1,276

TABLE 3.3
Alpha Center
Patient Records,
August 4–9, 2014

DAY	NUM	ART	AGE	TOWN	SEX	FIRST	INS	PHY	CHGE
1	1	815	23	1	2	1	1	2	120
1	2	817	64	2	2	2	1	2	120
1	3	819	34	1	2	3	1	2	96
1	4	820	45	1	2	2	1	2	124
1	5	822	17	6	2	1	1	2	120
1	6	822	56	4	1	1	8	2	288
1	7	830	19	6	1	2	2	2	120
1	8	833	7	4	1	3	1	2	96
1	9	855	56	1	2	1	1	2	120
1	10	905	32	2	2	1	1	2	128
1	11	910	34	4	1	2	1	2	120
1	12	915	23	1	2	1	9	1	80

(continued)

DAY	NUM	ART	AGE	TOWN	SEX	FIRST	INS	PHY	CHGE
1	13	925	21	7	2	2	9	1	80
1	14	1000	54	6	1	1	1	2	120
1	15	1012	51	1	1	1	8	2	276
1	16	1025	56	1	2	2	1	2	120
1	17	1105	49	4	1	2	1	2	126
1	18	1108	23	4	1	1	8	2	279
1	19	1203	45	2	1	2	8	2	243
1	20	1209	71	1	1	2	3	1	120
1	21	1215	71	1	1	2	3	2	140
1	22	1230	23	4	1	2	8	2	212
1	23	1245	28	1	1	2	8	2	230
1	24	1250	45	2	2	1	1	2	145
1	25	1255	47	1	2	2	1	1	120
1	26	1320	45	1	2	3	1	2	96
1	27	1345	22	2	1	1	8	2	201
1	28	1355	19	1	2	1	8	2	212
1	29	1420	34	1	2	2	9	2	80
1	30	1430	25	1	1	2	2	2	201
1	31	1435	68	1	1	2	3	2	201
1	32	1435	43	1	1	2	1	2	201
1	33	1512	3	2	1	1	1	2	120
1	34	1517	50	7	1	2	1	2	120
1	35	1537	63	2	1	2	1	2	209
1	36	1539	21	2	2	2	8	2	201
1	37	1545	56	1	1	2	9	1	80
1	38	1550	66	1	2	2	3	2	250
1	39	1555	19	1	1	1	8	2	270
1	40	1600	50	2	1	1	9	2	201

TABLE 3.3
Alpha Center
Patient Records,
August 4–9, 2014
(continued)

(continued)

DAY	NUM	ART	AGE	TOWN	SEX	FIRST	INS	PHY	CHGE
1	41	1600	43	2	1	2	9	2	201
1	42	1610	68	1	1	2	3	2	230
1	43	1625	50	2	1	2	9	2	350
1	44	1630	23	1	1	2	1	2	212
1	45	1645	18	1	1	1	1	2	208
1	46	1705	27	2	1	2	8	2	212
1	47	1740	45	2	2	2	1	2	240
1	48	1750	61	2	1	1	8	2	201
1	49	1800	57	4	2	1	1	2	120
1	50	1830	42	1	2	2	1	2	120
1	51	1830	40	1	1	1	1	2	120
1	52	1850	34	2	1	1	2	2	120
2	1	812	45	4	1	2	9	1	400
2	2	824	23	1	2	1	1	2	120
2	3	833	35	8	1	1	9	2	201
2	4	845	23	1	2	2	2	2	120
2	5	905	55	1	2	2	2	2	120
2	6	910	19	1	1	2	1	2	120
2	7	925	21	4	2	2	1	2	120
2	8	1010	33	2	1	1	8	2	201
2	9	1030	33	1	2	2	2	2	130
2	10	1055	33	2	1	1	9	1	275
2	11	1120	68	2	1	2	3	2	96
2	12	1205	61	1	2	2	8	2	201
2	13	1215	35	1	1	1	9	2	130
2	14	1215	4	1	1	1	1	2	120
2	15	1309	29	7	1	1	9	1	120
2	16	1310	25	6	2	1	1	2	120

(continued)

DAY	NUM	ART	AGE	TOWN	SEX	FIRST	INS	PHY	CHGE
2	17	1320	23	2	2	1	1	2	120
2	18	1400	55	8	1	1	2	2	130
2	19	1420	21	7	2	1	1	1	143
2	20	1421	21	1	2	1	8	2	240
2	21	1425	23	2	2	1	1	2	156
2	22	1507	50	2	2	2	2	2	138
2	23	1515	67	2	1	1	3	2	120
2	24	1555	4	1	1	3	2	2	145
2	25	1610	30	1	2	1	9	1	400
2	26	1620	24	2	1	1	1	2	120
2	27	1630	28	2	1	1	9	1	80
2	28	1650	37	1	1	2	8	2	201
2	29	1705	25	2	2	2	1	2	120
2	30	1720	22	1	2	1	1	2	120
2	31	1800	56	1	2	1	8	2	201
2	32	1810	77	1	1	2	9	1	300
2	33	1820	54	1	1	1	1	2	120
2	34	1825	32	1	1	2	1	2	120
3	1	801	24	2	1	1	1	2	120
3	2	810	45	1	1	2	8	2	201
3	3	825	2	4	1	1	1	2	120
3	4	835	34	1	1	1	1	2	120
3	5	845	66	1	2	2	3	2	150
3	6	915	44	1	1	1	9	1	80
3	7	920	26	4	1	1	9	1	300
3	8	950	23	1	2	1	1	2	120
3	9	1020	21	6	2	2	1	2	135
3	10	1040	25	1	1	1	1	2	120

TABLE 3.3
Alpha Center
Patient Records,
August 4–9, 2014
(continued)

(continued)

TABLE 3.3

Alpha Center Patient Records, August 4–9, 2014 (continued)

DAY	NUM	ART	AGE	TOWN	SEX	FIRST	INS	PHY	CHGE
3	11	1105	28	1	2	1	8	2	201
3	12	1130	69	1	2	2	3	2	120
3	13	1145	52	2	1	1	1	2	120
3	14	1200	50	2	2	2	8	2	156
3	15	1210	24	1	2	2	2	2	130
3	16	1245	21	7	2	3	1	2	135
3	17	1315	22	7	1	2	8	2	201
3	18	1315	21	2	2	2	8	2	250
3	19	1420	69	4	1	3	1	1	150
3	20	1450	23	4	1	2	8	2	201
3	21	1510	17	7	2	2	9	1	250
3	22	1520	14	2	1	1	8	2	201
3	23	1530	25	2	1	1	2	2	120
3	24	1600	31	2	2	3	1	2	96
3	25	1630	45	1	2	2	1	2	120
3	26	17151	55	1	1	2	1	2	120
3	27	1805	61	2	1	1	1	2	120
4	3	810	17	1	2	1	8	2	201
4	4	815	4	2	1	1	2	2	120
4	5	840	25	4	2	1	9	1	95
4	6	850	7	1	1	3	2	2	96
4	7	930	36	8	2	1	9	1	250
4	8	1000	44	2	2	1	9	1	400
4	9	1020	9	2	2	1	1	2	120
4	10	1050	44	1	2	2	8	2	201
4	11	1130	47	1	2	1	2	2	120
4	12	1205	34	4	1	1	8	2	201
4	13	1230	29	6	2	2	8	2	237

(continued)

DAY	NUM	ART	AGE	TOWN	SEX	FIRST	INS	PHY	CHGE
4	14	1245	28	1	2	3	2	2	140
4	15	1400	44	1	2	1	2	2	150
4	16	1430	12	1	1	2	1	2	120
4	17	1530	50	2	2	2	8	2	201
4	18	1600	23	1	1	1	1	2	120
4	19	1610	26	1	2	2	9	1	80
4	20	1620	39	2	2	2	9	1	300
4	21	1630	69	2	2	2	3	2	160
4	22	1730	30	1	2	2	1	2	145
4	23	1845	38	1	1	2	1	2	160
5	1	800	13	1	1	2	1	2	120
5	2	815	22	1	2	1	9	1	300
5	3	825	23	2	2	1	1	2	120
5	4	915	19	9	2	1	2	2	120
5	5	940	36	7	1	2	2	2	120
5	6	1000	45	2	1	1	9	1	300
5	7	1000	23	2	1	2	9	1	300
5	8	1045	60	1	1	3	2	2	96
5	9	1130	59	1	2	2	8	2	201
5	10	1215	52	4	1	1	2	2	120
5	11	1230	35	4	2	3	2	2	96
5	12	1240	21	7	2	1	1	2	120
5	13	1250	66	2	2	2	2	2	120
5	14	1310	45	2	2	1	8	2	201
5	15	1320	23	1	1	1	1	2	130
5	16	1350	21	1	2	1	1	2	150
5	17	1440	37	1	1	2	9	1	400
5	18	1510	40	6	2	2	9	1	400

TABLE 3.3
Alpha Center
Patient Records,
August 4–9, 2014
(continued)

(continued)

DAY	NUM	ART	AGE	TOWN	SEX	FIRST	INS	PHY	CHGE
5	19	1540	50	9	1	2	2	2	120
5	20	1620	66	8	2	2	3	2	130
5	21	1650	45	2	2	1	2	2	120
5	22	1715	54	2	2	2	8	2	201
5	23	1730	74	1	1	3	3	2	120
5	24	1730	3	1	2	2	2	2	120
5	25	1800	19	2	1	1	8	1	201
5	26	1820	47	2	2	1	8	1	201
5	27	1830	57	2	2	2	1	2	120
6	1	900	35	2	1	3	9	1	80
6	2	900	12	2	1	1	1	2	201
6	3	905	27	1	2	2	8	2	201
6	4	915	44	2	1	1	9	1	400
6	5	930	55	2	2	2	1	2	120
6	6	1000	23	3	1	1	1	2	120
6	7	1015	19	2	2	2	9	1	80
6	8	1015	7	7	2	2	9	2	201
6	9	1025	70	9	1	1	3	2	56
6	10	1040	24	8	1	1	9	1	80
6	11	1050	17	9	2	2	1	2	76
6	12	1100	19	2	2	2	1	2	76
6	13	1105	24	1	1	1	2	2	56
6	14	1115	16	2	2	2	2	2	76
6	15	1130	44	8	1	1	8	2	201
6	16	1145	48	2	2	1	8	2	201
6	17	1200	8	1	1	2	1	2	120
6	18	1215	76	1	1	2	3	2	130
6	19	1220	35	2	2	2	8	2	201

(continued)

DAY	NUM	ART	AGE	TOWN	SEX	FIRST	INS	PHY	CHGE
6	20	1230	50	1	1	1	9	1	80
6	21	1240	9	1	2	2	1	2	135
6	22	1240	23	2	1	3	1	2	120
6	23	1300	37	4	1	3	1	2	120
6	24	1315	61	5	2	2	1	2	120
6	25	1320	50	1	2	1	1	2	120
6	26	1340	72	2	1	2	3	2	120
Totals	189								$30,300

TABLE 3.3

Alpha Center Patient Records, August 4–9, 2014 (continued)

DAY = 1=Monday, 2= Tuesday, 3= Wednesday, 4= Thursday, 5= Friday, 6= Saturday
NUM = Arrival order (1 = first person to arrive)

ART = Arrival time   **AGE** = Age in years

TOWN:
1	Middleboro	6	Carterville
2	Mifflenville	7	Boalsburg
3	Jasper	8	Minortown
4	Harris City	9	Other
5	Statesville		

SEX 1 = male, 2 = female

FIRST = Is this your first ever visit to a PCS center?
1 Yes
2 No, and it is not a medically ordered return visit
3 No, it is a medically ordered return visit

INS = Insurance coverage/payment
1 Commercial insurance
2 Cash, check, or credit card
3 Medicare
8 Workers' compensation
9 Employer pays

PHY = Physical?
1 Yes
2 No

CHGE = Gross billed charges ($)

(This table can also be found online at ache.org/books/Middleboro.)

TABLE 3.4

Beta Center
Patient Records,
August 4–9, 2014

DAY	NUM	ART	AGE	TOWN	SEX	FIRST	INS	PHY	CHGE
1	1	800	44	3	2	2	8	2	385
1	2	810	32	3	1	1	1	2	135
1	3	810	45	3	2	1	8	2	370
1	4	845	66	3	1	1	3	2	96
1	5	845	21	5	1	1	8	2	380
1	6	900	7	9	2	3	1	2	150
1	7	915	34	3	2	1	8	2	350
1	8	930	51	3	2	1	8	2	360
1	9	945	59	3	2	1	1	2	180
1	10	1000	40	3	1	1	8	2	360
1	11	1005	23	5	1	2	9	1	300
1	12	1025	32	3	2	1	8	2	310
1	13	1035	40	5	2	2	1	2	160
1	14	1110	75	5	2	2	1	2	150
1	15	1150	22	3	1	1	9	1	300
1	16	1200	19	3	1	1	8	2	420
1	17	1015	56	3	2	2	9	1	150
1	18	1220	23	3	1	1	1	2	160
1	19	1310	34	3	1	1	8	2	310
1	20	1330	25	9	1	1	1	2	150
1	21	1410	49	3	2	2	9	1	150
1	22	1410	69	3	2	1	1	2	170
1	23	1430	70	9	2	2	3	2	135
1	24	1440	44	3	1	3	8	2	96
1	25	1450	25	3	1	1	8	2	325
1	26	1500	32	3	2	1	1	2	160
1	27	1605	37	9	2	2	8	2	375
1	28	1725	40	3	1	1	8	2	300

(continued)

DAY	NUM	ART	AGE	TOWN	SEX	FIRST	INS	PHY	CHGE
2	1	815	23	3	1	1	1	2	190
2	2	830	19	3	2	1	8	2	280
2	3	900	25	4	1	1	8	2	345
2	4	930	45	3	2	2	1	2	150
2	5	950	56	3	1	1	1	2	140
2	6	1015	8	9	1	1	1	2	120
2	7	1050	56	3	1	2	2	1	80
2	8	1120	23	9	1	1	1	1	80
2	9	1145	50	3	1	2	8	2	340
2	10	1215	56	3	2	1	8	2	350
2	11	1230	44	5	2	2	9	1	250
2	12	1250	47	3	1	1	8	2	285
2	13	11305	56	3	2	2	9	1	250
2	14	1310	23	9	2	1	1	2	130
2	15	1345	58	5	2	2	9	1	75
2	16	1400	44	5	1	1	1	2	150
2	17	1430	12	3	1	1	1	2	150
2	18	1500	40	3	2	1	8	2	315
2	19	1520	39	5	1	2	1	2	150
2	20	1520	47	9	1	2	8	1	250
2	21	1545	50	5	1	1	8	2	250
2	22	1610	46	5	2	1	9	1	250
2	23	1630	45	3	2	1	8	2	325
2	24	1645	23	3	1	2	1	2	140
2	25	1705	48	3	1	2	1	2	150
2	26	1730	32	3	1	2	1	2	140
3	1	800	23	3	1	1	1	2	160
3	2	845	19	3	1	1	1	2	160

TABLE 3.4
Beta Center
Patient Records,
August 4–9, 2014
(continued)

(continued)

TABLE 3.4
Beta Center
Patient Records,
August 4–9, 2014
(continued)

DAY	NUM	ART	AGE	TOWN	SEX	FIRST	INS	PHY	CHGE
3	3	920	44	3	2	2	8	2	275
3	4	1030	32	3	1	2	2	1	150
3	5	1110	50	5	1	2	8	2	350
3	6	1150	43	3	2	2	9	1	300
3	7	1200	50	3	2	2	1	2	150
3	8	1240	48	3	1	2	1	1	80
3	9	1250	50	5	1	1	8	2	350
3	10	1330	9	3	2	3	2	2	96
3	11	1600	45	3	2	1	1	2	160
3	12	1640	34	3	1	2	9	1	300
3	13	1700	56	3	1	1	9	1	300
3	14	1715	75	3	1	2	3	2	125
4	1	800	44	3	2	2	9	1	350
4	2	845	46	3	1	2	8	2	375
4	3	915	48	3	1	1	1	2	240
4	4	940	40	3	1	1	1	2	260
4	5	1035	23	9	1	1	8	2	350
4	6	1050	30	9	1	1	8	2	410
4	7	1130	50	3	1	1	1	2	160
4	8	1210	27	5	1	1	3	2	160
4	9	1230	22	9	1	1	3	2	120
4	10	1245	18	3	1	1	9	1	350
4	11	1320	23	3	2	2	1	2	140
4	12	1430	69	9	2	1	3	2	225
4	13	1510	45	9	1	2	9	1	250
4	14	1530	23	3	2	2	1	2	160
4	15	1610	12	3	2	3	1	2	150
4	16	1720	35	5	2	2	9	1	300

(continued)

DAY	NUM	ART	AGE	TOWN	SEX	FIRST	INS	PHY	CHGE
5	1	800	23	5	1	2	9	1	280
5	2	815	29	3	2	1	1	2	160
5	3	900	40	3	2	1	9	1	300
5	4	915	48	9	1	1	9	1	300
5	5	945	66	3	1	1	8	2	360
5	6	1015	45	2	1	1	1	1	150
5	7	1030	33	3	2	3	1	2	96
5	8	1140	21	5	1	1	9	1	300
5	9	1205	19	5	2	3	1	2	200
5	10	1210	45	3	2	2	8	2	340
5	11	1240	60	3	1	2	2	2	101
5	12	1250	55	3	2	1	8	2	320
5	13	1300	14	9	2	1	1	2	140
5	14	1320	23	3	2	1	9	1	300
5	15	1340	60	3	1	2	1	2	160
5	16	1400	69	3	1	2	3	2	120
5	17	1430	45	3	2	2	8	2	340
5	18	1500	4	5	1	3	1	2	96
5	19	1520	66	3	2	1	3	2	170
5	20	1540	19	5	2	2	9	1	240
5	21	1600	27	3	1	1	9	1	240
5	22	1700	44	3	2	2	1	2	160
5	23	1710	50	9	1	1	1	2	180
5	24	1710	20	5	1	1	8	2	310
5	25	1710	38	3	1	1	9	1	260
5	26	1740	34	9	2	2	1	2	140
6	1	910	5	3	1	1	1	2	160
6	2	930	23	3	2	2	1	2	170

TABLE 3.4
Beta Center Patient Records, August 4–9, 2014 (continued)

(continued)

TABLE 3.4
Beta Center
Patient Records,
August 4–9, 2014
(continued)

DAY	NUM	ART	AGE	TOWN	SEX	FIRST	INS	PHY	CHGE
6	3	1040	43	3	1	2	9	1	300
6	4	1050	44	3	2	1	9	1	150
6	5	1110	11	3	1	2	1	2	120
6	6	1120	48	9	2	2	1	2	150
6	7	1140	12	3	1	3	8	2	96
6	8	1215	12	3	1	2	9	1	200
6	9	1220	56	3	1	2	9	1	200
6	10	1300	60	5	1	2	9	1	200
6	11	1310	34	3	2	1	8	2	350
6	12	1330	63	3	1	2	3	2	140
Totals	**122**								**$27,177**

DAY = 1=Monday, 2= Tuesday, 3= Wednesday, 4= Thursday, 5= Friday, 6= Saturday
NUM = Arrival order (1 = first person to arrive)

ART = Arrival time   **AGE** = Age in years

TOWN: 1 Middleboro   6 Carterville
2 Mifflenville   7 Boalsburg
3 Jasper   8 Minortown
4 Harris City   9 Other
5 Statesville

SEX 1 = male, 2 = female

FIRST = Is this your first ever visit to a PCS center?
1 Yes
2 No, and it is not a medically ordered return visit
3 No, it is a medically ordered return visit

INS = Insurance coverage/payment
1 Commercial insurance
2 Cash, check, or credit card
3 Medicare
8 Workers' compensation
9 Employer pays

PHY = Physical?
1 Yes
2 No

CHGE = Gross billed charges ($)

(This table can also be found online at ache.org/books/Middleboro.)

RECORD	DATE	MD/ARNP	DAY	CTR	REVENUE ($)	VISITS
1	Sept 1	Holiday	1	1		
2	Sept 2	1	2	1	3,156	17
3	Sept 3	3	3	1	3,788	21
4	Sept 4	3	4	1	3,956	23
5	Sept 5	1	5	1	3,059	24
6	Sept 6	11	6	1	3,076	19
7	Sept 8	1	1	1	3,044	22
8	Sept 9	1	2	1	3,657	34
9	Sept 10	3	3	1	4,366	20
10	Sept 11	3	4	1	4,381	25
11	Sept 12	4	5	1	3,547	38
12	Sept 13	11	6	1	3,148	16
13	Sept 15	1	1	1	3,008	23
14	Sept 16	1	2	1	3,005	18
15	Sept 17	3	3	1	3,976	21
16	Sept 18	3	4	1	3,740	19
17	Sept 19	4	5	1	3,547	30
18	Sept 20	11	6	1	3,005	20
19	Sept 22	1	1	1	3,259	32
20	Sept 23	1	2	1	3,051	22
21	Sept 24	3	3	1	3,906	18
22	Sept 25	3	4	1	3,856	22
23	Sept 26	4	5	1	3,944	24
24	Sept 27	11	6	1	3,452	20
25	Sept 29	1	1	1	3,056	20
26	Sept 30	1	2	1	3,067	23
27	Oct 1	3	3	1	3,010	23
28	Oct 2	3	4	1	2,840	18
29	Oct 3	5	5	1	3,049	20
30	Oct 4	11	6	1	1,599	10
31	Oct 6	1	1	1	6,559	42
32	Oct 7	1	2	1	3,769	21
33	Oct 8	3	3	1	3,276	20
34	Oct 9	3	4	1	3,806	20
35	Oct 10	4	5	1	3,051	18
36	Oct 11	11	6	1	3,028	20
37	Oct 13	1	1	1	5,278	33
38	Oct 14	1	2	1	4,650	28
39	Oct 15	3	3	1	3,920	20

TABLE 3.5

Revenue
Generation by
Physician, Center,
Day of Week,
September 1–
November 29, 2014

(continued)

TABLE 3.5

Revenue
Generation by
Physician, Center,
Day of Week,
September 1–
November 29, 2014
(continued)

RECORD	DATE	MD/ARNP	DAY	CTR	REVENUE ($)	VISITS
40	Oct 16	3	4	1	2,534	14
41	Oct 17	5	5	1	4,020	28
42	Oct 18	11	6	1	3,699	24
43	Oct 20	1	1	1	4,460	36
44	Oct 21	1	2	1	4,739	28
45	Oct 22	3	3	1	4,230	22
46	Oct 23	3	4	1	3,288	19
47	Oct 24	4	5	1	3,805	25
48	Oct 25	11	6	1	3,397	22
49	Oct 27	1	1	1	5,520	39
50	Oct 28	1	2	1	4,367	28
51	Oct 29	3	3	1	3,650	20
52	Oct 30	3	4	1	3,090	18
53	Oct 31	4	5	1	3,001	20
54	Nov 1	11	6	1	1,145	10
55	Nov 3	1	1	1	5,350	35
56	Nov 4	1	2	1	2,768	15
57	Nov 5	3	3	1	3,587	21
58	Nov 6	3	4	1	4,879	26
59	Nov 7	5	5	1	2,757	19
60	Nov 8	11	6	1	1,036	10
61	Nov 10	1	1	1	5,567	31
62	Nov 11	1	2	1	2,586	17
63	Nov 12	3	3	1	5,980	32
64	Nov 13	3	4	1	4,771	24
65	Nov 14	4	5	1	2,061	14
66	Nov 15	13	6	1	2,212	22
67	Nov 17	1	1	1	5,789	35
68	Nov 18	1	2	1	3,879	23
69	Nov 19	3	3	1	5,879	31
70	Nov 20	3	4	1	4,244	24
71	Nov 21	5	5	1	2,959	17
72	Nov 22	11	6	1	2,055	15
73	Nov 24	1	1	1	4,789	30
74	Nov 25	1	2	1	4,444	25
75	Nov 26	3	3	1	5,546	32
76	Nov 27	Holiday	4	1		
77	Nov 28	9	5	1	4,007	30
78	Nov 29	11	6	1	2,335	16

(continued)

RECORD	DATE	MD/ARNP	DAY	CTR	REVENUE ($)	VISITS
79	Sept 1	Holiday	1	2		
80	Sept 2	2	2	2	5,157	25
81	Sept 3	6	3	2	4,286	14
82	Sept 4	6	4	2	4,367	16
83	Sept 5	7	5	2	4,156	17
84	Sept 6	13	6	2	1,956	10
85	Sept 8	2	1	2	6,648	30
86	Sept 9	2	2	2	5,978	29
87	Sept 10	6	3	2	4,934	20
88	Sept 11	6	4	2	2,166	12
89	Sept 12	7	5	2	4,305	16
90	Sept 13	13	6	2	1,510	9
91	Sept 15	2	1	2	6,250	28
92	Sept 16	2	2	2	4,850	20
93	Sept 17	6	3	2	3,956	18
94	Sept 18	7	4	2	4,707	20
95	Sept 19	8	5	2	3,958	18
96	Sept 20	13	6	2	1,941	10
97	Sept 22	2	1	2	5,790	28
98	Sept 23	2	2	2	4,415	20
99	Sept 24	6	3	2	3,083	14
100	Sept 25	8	4	2	3,546	16
101	Sept 26	8	5	2	4,026	16
102	Sept 27	12	6	2	1,850	12
103	Sept 29	2	1	2	4,890	24
104	Sept 30	2	2	2	3,827	18
105	Oct 1	5	3	2	4,080	18
106	Oct 2	5	4	2	3,080	15
107	Oct 3	8	5	2	2,044	9
108	Oct 4	13	6	2	830	4
109	Oct 6	2	1	2	4,560	20
110	Oct 7	2	2	2	4,050	20
111	Oct 8	5	3	2	4,069	20
112	Oct 9	5	4	2	3,827	18
113	Oct 10	6	5	2	1,566	11
114	Oct 11	13	6	2	1,209	6
115	Oct 13	2	1	2	4,038	19
116	Oct 14	2	2	2	4,740	20
117	Oct 15	5	3	2	3,567	17

TABLE 3.5

Revenue Generation by Physician, Center, Day of Week, September 1–November 29, 2014 (continued)

(continued)

RECORD	DATE	MD/ARNP	DAY	CTR	REVENUE ($)	VISITS
118	Oct 16	5	4	2	5,035	18
119	Oct 17	6	5	2	3,077	15
120	Oct 18	13	6	2	1,518	8
121	Oct 20	2	1	2	5,734	22
122	Oct 21	2	2	2	3,657	19
123	Oct 22	5	3	2	3,256	20
124	Oct 23	5	4	2	3,070	13
125	Oct 24	6	5	2	3,058	12
126	Oct 25	12	6	2	1,656	8
127	Oct 27	2	1	2	5,020	22
128	Oct 28	2	2	2	4,640	20
129	Oct 29	5	3	2	2,748	15
130	Oct 30	5	4	2	2,978	14
131	Oct 31	6	5	2	2,007	9
132	Nov 1	13	6	2	1,205	6
133	Nov 3	2	1	2	3,557	17
134	Nov 4	2	2	2	4,047	15
135	Nov 5	6	3	2	3,344	18
136	Nov 6	6	4	2	4,289	20
137	Nov 7	8	5	2	3,756	14
138	Nov 8	13	6	2	1,034	4
139	Nov 10	2	1	2	4,420	30
140	Nov 11	2	2	2	4,510	16
141	Nov 12	6	3	2	3,089	16
142	Nov 13	6	4	2	3,837	15
143	Nov 14	8	5	2	4,730	17
144	Nov 15	13	6	2	1,856	10
145	Nov 17	2	1	2	4,298	21
146	Nov 18	2	2	2	3,587	12
147	Nov 19	6	3	2	2,689	13
148	Nov 20	6	4	2	4,856	22
149	Nov 21	7	5	2	3,962	14
150	Nov 22	13	6	2	1,091	10
151	Nov 24	2	1	2	5,029	24
152	Nov 25	2	2	2	2,538	12
153	Nov 26	6	3	2	2,177	12
154	Nov 27	Holiday	4	2		
155	Nov 28	9	5	2	2,002	8
156	Nov 29	13	6	2	1,053	5

(continued)

CODES For Table 3.5		
MD/ARNP	**Day**	**Center**
1	B. Casey	Monday	Alpha
2	M. Welby	Tuesday	Beta
3	S. Tobias	Wednesday	
4	J. Smooth	Thursday	
5	R. Hottle	Friday	
6	L. Cytesmath	Saturday	
7	J. Withers		
8	L. Jones		
9	M. Foxx		
10	M. Majors		
11	C. Withers, ARNP		
12	J. Jones, ARNP		
13	G Mattox, ARNP		

Revenue = Total gross billed charges
Visits = Number of paying patients

TABLE 3.5

Revenue Generation by Physician, Center, Day of Week, September 1– November 29, 2014 (continued)

(This table can also be found online at ache.org/books/Middleboro.)

TABLE 3.6
Statement of
Operations ($)

	2014	2013	2012	2011	2010
Revenue					
Patient services, gross	2,246,188	1,993,211	1,918,406	1,696,999	1,690,252
Contractual alllowances	179,695	159,457	153,472	135,760	135,220
Patient revenue, net	2,066,493	1,833,754	1,764,934	1,561,239	1,555,032
Other revenue	18,520	22,463	22,252	23,595	23,684
Total revenue	**2,085,013**	**1,856,217**	**1,787,186**	**1,584,834**	**1,578,716**
Expenses					
Salaries and wages	1,131,608	1,001,556	982,450	839,229	838,226
Staff benefits	392,301	310,482	294,735	243,376	234,703
Administrative expenses	18,330	17,339	10,494	10,056	9,562
Advertising	3,000	3,400	3,856	3,003	2,340
Collection fees	1,267	845	342	659	589
Computer support	21,556	31,443	34,256	35,378	25,398
Consultants	1,529	1,270	948	805	355
Equipment leases	4,100	4,100	4,100	1,800	1,800
Insurance	28,100	24,100	24,100	18,560	24,100
Laboratory	44,870	45,292	42,550	44,691	39,254
Laundry and housekeeping	12,830	12,256	8,156	3,440	2,440
Legal/audit	8,450	8,450	8,450	7,850	7,850
Medical supplies	61,450	58,220	57,354	58,556	28,340
Office supplies	18,437	29,348	28,420	28,556	28,360
Printing and postage	10,122	9,450	9,014	3,588	2,013
Professional fees	23,955	23,425	23,302	23,884	24,885
Rent	78,500	78,750	58,900	58,900	58,900
Repairs and maintenance	3,167	2,966	1,529	2,349	3,620
Telephone	10,315	7,495	6,519	2,550	2,044
Utilities	18,925	16,800	13,560	13,720	13,900
Depreciation	72,556	70,449	70,383	68,363	79,262
Bad debt expenses	8,437	5,629	4,303	3,494	3,102
Total expenses	**1,973,805**	**1,763,065**	**1,687,721**	**1,472,807**	**1,431,043**
Income (loss) before taxes	111,208	93,152	99,465	112,027	147,673
Federal and state taxes	44,483	37,261	39,786	44,811	59,069
Income (loss) after taxes	**66,725**	**55,891**	**59,679**	**67,216**	**88,604**

(This table can also be found online at ache.org/books/Middleboro.)

	2014	2013	2012	2011	2010
Assets					
Current					
Cash, operating	153,449	163,035	86,999	76,223	84,550
Accounts receivable	139,385	134,450	131,560	130,455	168,455
Inventory	3,339	4,125	5,233	28,734	30,335
Prepaid expenses	3,078	4,565	4,021	5,688	8,944
Total current assets	**299,251**	**306,175**	**227,813**	**241,100**	**292,284**
Investments	368,825	341,010	405,903	353,628	314,040
Property and equipment					
Equipment and leasehold improvements, gross	1,197,602	1,125,046	1,054,597	984,214	915,851
Less accumulated depreciation	645,239	572,683	502,234	431,851	363,488
Equipment and leasehold improvements, net	552,363	552,363	552,363	552,363	552,363
Total assets	**1,220,439**	**1,199,548**	**1,186,079**	**1,147,091**	**1,158,687**
Liabilities and net assets					
Current liabilities					
Accounts payable	49,668	13,534	13,796	10,455	77,454
Accrued expenses	29,000	27,387	30,100	45,662	23,145
Accrued payroll taxes	2,134	945	823	1,126	569
Total current liabilities	80,802	41,866	44,719	57,243	101,168
Long-term liabilities					
Notes payable	0	84,770	124,339	132,506	167,393
Total liabilities	**80,802**	**126,636**	**169,058**	**189,749**	**268,561**

TABLE 3.7
Balance Sheet for Fiscal Year Ending December 31 ($)

(continued)

TABLE 3.7

Balance Sheet for Fiscal Year Ending December 31 (continued)

	2014	2013	2012	2011	2010
Net assets					
Common stock note[1]					
Authorized and issued	720,000	720,000	720,000	720,000	720,000
Cumulative operating gain/ (deficit) after taxes	371,637	352,912	297,021	237,342	170,126
Dividends payable	48,000				
Net assets	**1,139,637**	**1,072,912**	**1,017,021**	**957,342**	**890,126**
Net assets and liabilities	**1,220,439**	**1,199,548**	**1,186,079**	**1,147,091**	**1,158,687**

NOTE: 1. Common stock: $12 par, 60,000 authorized and issued.

(This table can also be found online at ache.org/books/Middleboro.)

TABLE 3.8

Compensation for the 12 Months Ending December 31, 2014 ($)

	Salary	Benefits	Total
President	40,000	14,400	54,400
Medical director	20,000	7,200	27,200
subtotal	60,000	21,600	81,600
Clinical staff			
Casey	114,400	41,184	155,584
Welby	116,600	41,976	158,576
Tobias	125,400	45,144	170,544
Smooth	77,000	27,720	104,720
Hottle	52,800	19,008	71,808

(continued)

	Salary	Benefits	Total
Cytesmath	52,800	19,008	71,808
Withers	11,000	2,420	13,420
Jones	7,700	1,694	9,394
Foxx	5,500	1,210	6,710
Withers, ARNP	10,000	2,200	12,200
Jones, ARNP	4,000	880	4,880
Mattox, ARNP	12,000	2,640	14,640
Others	3,100	682	3,782
subtotal	592,300	205,766	798,066
Professional services			
Medical assistants	92,280	33,221	125,501
Receptionists	86,128	31,006	117,134
Others	2,400	528	2,928
subtotal	180,808	64,755	245,563
Administrative services			
Director of nursing and quality	64,000	23,040	87,040
Business manager	62,500	22,500	85,000
Business office staff (4 FTE)	120,000	43,200	163,200
Others	52,000	11,440	63,440
subtotal	298,500	100,180	398,680
Total	**1,131,608**	**392,301**	**1,523,909**

TABLE 3.8
Compensation for the 12 Months Ending December 31, 2014 (continued)

Patient Revenue	2,424,000
Deductions	198,768
Net revenue	**2,225,232**
Expenses	
Salaries and wages	1,181,200
Staff benefits	425,230
Administrative expenses	21,500
Advertising	3,000
Collection fees	1,800
Consultants	3,750
Computer support	34,000
Equipment leases	4,100
Insurance	28,100
Laboratory	49,000
Laundry and housekeeping	13,500
Legal/audit	8,450
Medical supplies	64,750
Printing and postage	11,000
Professional fees	28,000
Rent	78,500
Repairs	3,500
Telephone	11,000
Utilities	19,200
Depreciation	73,000
Bad debt expenses	10,400
Total expenses	**2,072,980**

(continued)

Income (loss) before taxes	152,252
Taxes	60,901
Income (loss) after taxes	91,351

TABLE 3.9
Proposed
Operational
Budget for 2015 ($)
(continued)

NOTE:

Budget parameters	Alpha	Beta	Total
Visits, budgeted	7,500	5,100	12,600
Average revenue per visit ($) with no increased basic visit fee	160	240	

(This table can also be found online at ache.org/books/Middleboro.)

	2014	2013	2012	2011	2010
Middleboro Community Hospital ED	210	200	190	180	180
Webster Hospital ED (Quick Med)[1]	140	140	140	125	125
Convenient Med Care, Capital City[1]	125	125	125	115	115
Capital City General ED	180	180	170	150	150
Medical Associates[1]	125	125	125	115	115
PCS[1]	120	110	104	99	94

TABLE 3.10
Market Analysis of
Basic Visit Charges
as of July 1 ($)

1 = Comparisons based on CPT 99202

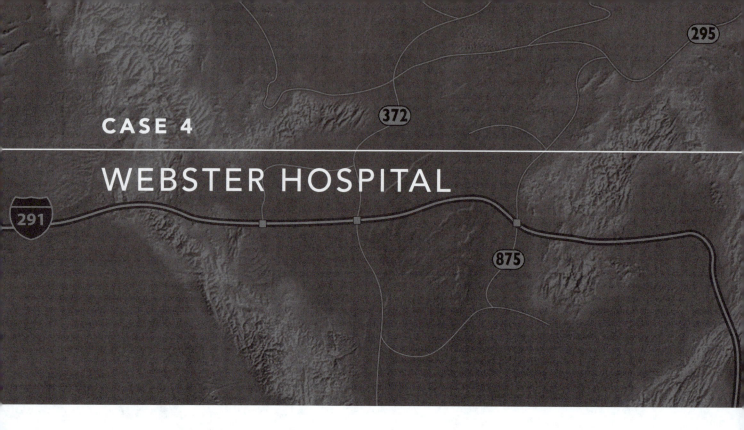

CASE 4

WEBSTER HOSPITAL

Webster Hospital was founded in 1930 as a short-term, general, acute-care nonprofit hospital. It currently is licensed to operate 105 inpatient beds and has met all conditions necessary for its services to be covered by Medicaid, Medicare, and Blue Cross and Blue Shield. The hospital and a for-profit organization jointly owned by the hospital and members of the medical staff constitute the Webster Health System. The American Osteopathic Association accredits the hospital; Webster is an affiliate member of Osteopathic Hospitals of America, Inc. (OHA), headquartered in Capital City. Current hospital services as reported by the American Hospital Association include:

- Airborne infection isolation room
- Auxiliary organization
- Birthing room, LDR room, LDRP Room
- Blood donor center
- Breast cancer screening/ mammograms
- Adult cardiology services

- Endoscopic retrograde
- Enrollment assistance services
- Electron beam computed tomography
- Extracorporeal shock wave lithotripter
- Health fair

- Physical rehabilitation outpatient services
- CT scanner
- Diagnostic radioisotope facility
- Magnetic resonance imaging
- Full-field digital mammography

- Case management
- Chaplaincy/pastoral care
- Chemotherapy
- Children's wellness program
- Community health reporting
- Community health status assessment
- Community health status-based service planning
- Community outreach
- Complementary and alternative medicine
- Computer-assisted orthopedic surgery
- Crisis prevention
- Emergency department
- Enabling services
- Palliative care program
- Endoscopic ultrasound
- Ablation of Barrett's esophagus

- Community health education
- Health screening
- Hospital-based outpatient care center services
- Immunization program
- Medical surgical intensive care services
- Mobile health services
- Nutritional programs
- Obstetrics
- Occupational health services
- Oncology services
- Orthopedic services
- Other special care
- Outpatient surgery
- Patient-controlled analgesia
- Patient education center
- Patient representative services

- Multislice spiral computed tomography, <64-slice CT
- Single photon emission computerized tomography
- Ultrasound
- Fertility clinic
- Genetic testing/counseling
- Robotic surgery
- Sleep center
- Social work services
- Sports medicine
- Support groups
- Tobacco treatment/ cessation program
- Transportation to health services
- Urgent care center
- Virtual colonoscopy
- Women's health center/ services

OSTEOPATHIC HOSPITALS OF AMERICA

Headquartered in Capital City, OHA is a nonprofit corporation that provides tertiary care and includes a regional network of 18 affiliated community nonprofit osteopathic hospitals under a master board of directors. Harry Swift is the chief executive officer (CEO) of OHA.

OHA began in 1990 to provide corporate direction and control for osteopathic hospitals in the region. Individual hospitals elect to affiliate in the system and retain their independent corporate status. Annually, the board of OHA votes to retain an affiliate member and has the ability to sever the affiliation contract with 12 months' notice. Under a formal affiliation contract (renewed annually) a hospital agrees:

◆ to retain its membership for at least three years and to elect 1 person to the OHA board of directors,

◆ to provide consulting and/or active privileges to all qualified physicians recommended to it by OHA,

- ◆ to record all patient care information using the OHA medical records system and share this information in abstract form with OHA,

- ◆ to purchase all supply items (medical and nonmedical) and durable medical equipment through OHA,

- ◆ to provide OHA with its draft revenue and expense budget for the next fiscal year and bring to its board all comments on this budget rendered by OHA,

- ◆ to provide OHA with a first option for purchase if the hospital decides to change its ownership status, and

- ◆ to pay OHA an annual affiliation fee of 0.005 percent of its gross charges or $1,000,000, whichever is less.

In return for this affiliation, hospitals receive a series of services and benefits at no additional cost:

- ◆ Board education

- ◆ Development of the hospital's strategic plan and quality assurance system

- ◆ Access to capital for projects approved by OHA at prime rate plus 0.2 percent

- ◆ Continuing medical education

- ◆ Consulting services related to electronic health records, financial management, human resources administration, health benefit surveys, and new service development

- ◆ Tele-Med Services—a high-speed voice and video communications link between the attending physicians at an affiliated hospital and physicians at Osteopathic Medical Center (OMC)

- ◆ Regional and community specific advertising services

Under the affiliation agreement, a hospital also may hire (i.e., lease) a CEO from OHA (at cost); use OHA service-marked services, such as Quick Med; and use (at cost) OMC AIR EVAC.

OHA is organized into three divisions:

Osteopathic Medical Center

Located in Capital City, this 210-bed medical center provides a full range of acute and tertiary care services. OMC is a nonprofit corporation and a designated teaching hospital offering approved residencies in most medical specialties. OMC is also a Level I Trauma Center. Samuel Gilbert, DO, is president of OMC. Medical interns and residents visit Webster Hospital regularly as part of their community medicine training. This past month, OMC alerted member hospitals (confidentially) that the governor's office is working with other states on model legislation to limit hospital costs. One model being considered limits annual hospital spending increases to the annual increase in gross state product.

OHA Hospital Services, Inc.

OHA Hospital Services, Inc. (OHAHS) is a nonprofit corporation also located in Capital City. It provides services to OMC and all OHA-affiliated hospitals. Garrett Fulerman is president. Current services include the following:

◆   Supply chain management

◆   Retirement services plan

◆   Hospital risk management programs

◆   OHA health services consulting

◆   OHA outplacement and recruiting service

◆   Capital financing services

◆   Meaningful use advisory services

◆   Electronic health and medical record systems

OHA Ventures, Inc.

OHA Ventures, Inc. (OHAV) is a for-profit corporation located in Capital City and headed by Jane Ramirez. Currently OHAV specializes in managing medical groups. It also owns and operates medical office buildings. Three years ago OHAV began a joint purchase and management program under which an affiliate OHA member hospital and OHAV purchase and manage individual medical practices. Webster was one of the first OHA affiliate members to participate in this program.

History and Physical Structure of Webster Hospital

Webster Hospital was originally built to house 70 inpatient beds and expanded in 1982 to accommodate 105 beds. Today, the hospital operates 95 inpatient beds. The facility is a three-floor brick structure and has been modernized over the years. It currently meets or exceeds all building standards. The hospital is located on a 246-acre campus in southeastern Middleboro, adjacent to the interstate highway. A modernization program completed three years ago provides this hospital with an attractive physical plant arranged for the efficient delivery of modern medicine. This recent modernization also expanded maternity services so that when possible all maternity services—including delivery—are provided in the mother's room.

Adjacent to the hospital are structures originally built as homes that are now owned by the hospital. These homes are rented as office space for 12 members of the medical staff. All of the other land on the hospital campus is undeveloped.

Founded by EW Webster, DO, in 1930, Webster Hospital has had close ties with OMC in Capital City even before the development of OHA. Prior to arriving in Middleboro in 1929, Dr. Webster had been a senior physician at OMC. In 1929 Dr. Webster began a community campaign to found an alternative hospital. He served as the first superintendent of the hospital and was successful in establishing osteopathic medicine in this region. The Webster family continues to financially support this hospital. Over the past 20 years, his sons and grandsons have continued to enhance the hospital's endowment.

Since its inception, this hospital has tended to mirror the characteristics of its medical staff. The majority of the hospital's active medical staff provides primary care. Patients needing more sophisticated operations, tests, or medical care are referred or transferred to OMC or served by consulting members of the Webster Hospital medical staff, who travel to Webster Hospital when needed. Webster Hospital maintains a helicopter pad to permit the rapid transfer of emergency patients to OMC by the OMC AIR EVAC. OMC AIR EVAC has also been used to bring physicians from OMC to Webster Hospital as needed. Air travel time from Webster Hospital to OMC is approximately 16 minutes. When weather conditions do not permit air transfer to and from OMC, patients can be transferred to Middleboro Community Hospital or, by ambulance, to OMC.

Since 1930, relations with Middleboro Community Hospital have been strained. As examples, the joint venture corporation owned in partnership with Middleboro Community Hospital for shared laundry services was dissolved 12 years ago. Middleboro Community Hospital elected a provision in the original 1965 agreement to buy Webster Hospital's share of the joint service corporation, even though Webster Hospital wished for the joint venture corporation to be retained. At that time of forced sale, Middleboro Community Hospital indicated its need for laundry services could only be met if it fully owned the laundry corporation. While Middleboro Community Hospital did offer to provide laundry services to Webster Hospital on an annual contract, Webster Hospital determined it would be more efficient if it reestablished its own service. Another example involves the termination of the joint education agreement with Middleboro Community Hospital ten years ago. Under this agreement, continuing education for staff was centralized to serve both institutions. The sole remaining cooperative agreement between the two hospitals involves oncology. Under this agreement, ambulatory cancer treatment is available at Middleboro Community Hospital for patients under the care of a DO. This provision was required by the state when the Certificate of Need was originally issued to Middleboro Community Hospital for this service.

It should also be noted that a formal joint committee of the boards of each hospital explored merger of the two hospitals 22 years ago. Although the idea was supported by both CEOs, the committee concluded that merger would not be feasible. Since that time Webster Hospital and Middleboro Community Hospital have had minimal contact and exist in an increasingly competitive environment.

When Webster Hospital signed the original affiliation agreement with OHA in 2000, the CEO and board chairman at Middleboro Community Hospital wrote a letter, published in the *Middleboro Sentinel*, indicating how disappointed they were that a community hospital in their town was now going to be "directed by a medical center outside the community" and that they wished they had known that "Webster Hospital obviously needed help to continue to provide quality patient care at a reasonable price."

GOVERNANCE AND ORGANIZATION

Webster Hospital's board of trustees is composed of eight individuals. The 100 incorporators, chosen by the board's nominating committee, elect trustees. Trustees are elected for four-year terms with the stipulation that no individual may serve longer than two consecutive terms. Current board officers are:

Name	Board Position	Occupation	Residence
Daniel Will	Chairman (2)*	Attorney, Will & Associates	Middleboro
Harlan Crowe	Vice chairman (3)	President, Farmers and Merchants Bank	Mifflenville
Janice Nice	Secretary (4)	Director of human resources, US Parts, Inc.	Jasper
Mary Bond	Treasurer (1)	Stockbroker (retired)	Boalsburg
Steve Hickery	At-large (1)	Agricultural Business	Statesville
Joan Meyer	At-large (2)	Vice president, Finance, River Industries	Middleboro
Philip Werner, DO	At-large (3)	Physician	Middleboro
Eric Martin	At-large (4)	President and CEO, Carlstead Rayon	Middleboro

* Indicates years remaining on term of office. Note that trustees Will and Bond are currently serving their second consecutive term and cannot be reelected.

Standing committees of the board are:

Executive	All board officers
Finance	Crowe (chair), Bond, Martin
Joint Conference	Will, Morgan, Masterman (CEO)
Long-Range Planning	All trustees
Medical Staffing/Credentials	Werner (chair), Meyer, Hickery
Nominating	Nice (chair), Crowe, Martin
Quality Assurance	Myers (chair), Will, Heart

The board of trustees meets monthly. The executive committee meets twice a month. Other committees meet as needed, usually monthly. Every December the board of trustees in cooperation with the hospital auxiliary sponsors the Holiday Ball at the Middleboro Golf Club as a hospital fund-raising event.

SENIOR MANAGEMENT TEAM
President and CEO

Janice Masterman, RN, has held this position for the last 19 years. Her career at the hospital has spanned more than 30 years and has included service in the nursing department and the business office. She was born in Middleboro and is a registered nurse, having graduated from a diploma nursing school in Capital City. Since returning to Middleboro 30 years ago, she completed her undergraduate degree in health administration and her master of business administration at the State University on a part-time basis. After serving four years as a charge nurse, she requested transfer to the business office to gain experience in fiscal management. At the time of her appointment as interim president, she was the hospital's controller.

Combining a keen sensitivity for both clinical and administrative matters, Masterman has, over the past 19 years, led the hospital through crisis after crisis. She is well liked by all employees and on a first name basis with most. She is known for her ability to delegate tasks and make difficult administrative decisions. She appears to have the respect of the medical staff. She was appointed to her position on a permanent basis two years after being appointed on an interim basis when a national search yielded no other qualified candidate.

On numerous occasions she has received recognition from the board. For example, the board officially commended her for the leadership she demonstrated concerning the affiliation agreement with OMC. Prior to this contractual agreement, relationships with OMC had evolved but had not been covered by a formal contract. Since the affiliation was ratified, Webster Hospital has been able to receive multiple benefits and embarked upon a program of physician recruitment with an emphasis in family practice. Recently, OHA provided Webster the consulting services to establish a physician hospital organization as part of Webster's redefinition as Webster Health System.

When recently interviewed Masterman indicated her high level of satisfaction with the relationship that emerged with OHA and indicated that through this relationship Webster Hospital had solved its emergency department staffing problem, established Quick Med as a walk-in primary care service, and expanded its medical staff.

Over the past five years, Webster Hospital has adjusted to changing inpatient utilization patterns. Masterman indicated that the advice and guidance furnished by OHC was instrumental to her hospital's continued success and its decision to use downsizing as the opportunity to offer private rooms for medical/surgical patients.

Over the years, OMC has advised Webster Hospital to close its dedicated orthopedic unit and serve orthopedic patients with fewer medical/surgical inpatient beds. She was also advised to reduce staffing only through retirements and resignations and not terminate any employees; if necessary, employees would be retained for essential duties in the hospital. At the same time, OHC advised Webster Hospital to slowly increase the size of it maternity service. Ms. Masterman indicated that this advice has been instrumental in the current success enjoyed by her hospital.

Masterman chairs the hospital's "meaningful use" taskforce. She reports that the hospital was the first hospital in the county to qualify under this program and continues to receive maximum awards for meeting and exceeding all federal requirements.

When asked about the success of past plans and strategies, she mentioned board education: "My board knows good business practice. The educational programs they have participated in that have been sponsored by OHA provide them the ability to translate these business practices into sound plans for the hospital. A great deal of our success rests with a knowledgeable board. For someone like me, this is a great board to work for." Masterman also indicated that she has officially notified the board that she will be retiring in 12 months but was willing to continue as the Webster Hospital representative on the board of OHA and/or as a trustee of Webster Hospital.

Masterman is a Fellow of the American College of Healthcare Executives (ACHE). She is also a published author, a frequent speaker at local civic events, and an elected member of the Middleboro School Board. The governor recently nominated Masterman as one of the top 25 Women Health Leaders in the state.

Vice President for Administrative Services/Chief Financial Officer

Steve Swisher, a certified public accountant, has served as vice president and chief financial officer for 14 years. He holds an undergraduate degree in accounting and a master of business administration from a midwestern university. Prior to his affiliation with this hospital, he was a senior fiscal analyst with Blue Cross and Blue Shield in Capital City. He is a member of the Healthcare Financial Management Association (HFMA). He reports to the president and has responsibility for the following departments:

◆ Admitting

◆ Business office

◆ Central supply

◆ Housekeeping

◆ Laundry

◆ Maintenance

◆ Medical records

◆ Personnel

◆ Purchasing

◆ Security

◆ Telecommunications

When recently interviewed he indicated that he had just returned from signing a five-year contract to provide laundry services for the county nursing home. Last year, Webster Hospital began searching for clients to use its excess laundry capacity, caused by the decrease in inpatient days. Swisher said that aside from good business, this contract would keep the hospital's laundry service an efficient operation with its current level of staffing.

Swisher is considered a statewide expert on hospital reimbursement policies and practices. He lecturers at State University and is on numerous statewide panels involved with the health insurance industry. He also stated that he felt the personnel department was getting to be too complex, and it will need professional leadership, especially after Masterman retires. According to Swisher, personnel has become "an almost full-time job." He also indicated that the heavy investment the hospital made in a fully integrated management and clinical information system four years ago was showing results. He said that the hospital and medical staff joint continuous quality improvement (CQI) program has been successful because of the information reported by this system. He cited the hospital and medical staff's ability to shorten average length of stay as a direct benefit associated with this system.

When asked about the future, Swisher was optimistic. He indicated that Masterman would be very hard to replace and that the hospital's inpatient capacity has gotten about as small as it should—"Too much smaller and it will become less efficient." As a result, he advocates a competitive strategy that targets capturing ambulatory and inpatient market share historically served by Middleboro Community Hospital. He noted that the hospital's relationship with its staff, including the medical staff, was positive. "They know our needs, we know theirs, and we are committed to joint success."

Under Swisher's leadership and strong support from OHA, Webster Hospital launched its electronic health record system five years ago. After limited pilot testing, the system, which includes order entry, became operational in 2010. Any medical practice owned by Webster Hospital is also online. For all other medical practices access to the system requires that the medical practice purchase or lease the needed hardware from OHA/Webster Hospital. Technical oversight of the system is provided by a private contractor and OHAHS, Inc. When asked, Swisher responded that the hospital did not need an additional chief information systems officer at this time. "Our current arrangement seems to be working. We have the needed expertise in OHAHS and the contractor is responsive to our needs."

At the last management team meeting Swisher reported that the 2014 CMS calculated case mix index for Webster Hospital was 1.3245. Case mix index is a proxy measure for patient acuity—the higher the number, the more complex the patient population. Webster's number is low compared with other hospitals, even of its type, nationally, but the increase suggests that the hospital is also having to deal with a sicker patient population. According to Swisher, "We are like most hospitals. Our index has increased slightly each year over the past five years."

Vice President for Professional Services

Ellen Wilgus has been employed by Webster Hospital for 11 years and has served as vice president for professional services for the past seven years. Prior to her appointment as vice president, she was director of the physical therapy department. She holds an undergraduate degree in physical therapy from the State University. She has served as president of the state chapter of the American Physical Therapy Association and remains active in professional organizations related to physical therapy and rehabilitation. Wilgus reports to the president and has responsibility for the following departments:

◆ Anesthesiology

◆ Dietary

◆ Laboratory

◆ Pharmacy

◆ Physical therapy

◆ Radiology

◆ Respiratory therapy

◆ Social services

When interviewed, Wilgus expressed concern over the ever-increasing complexities associated with hospital management. She also indicated that she felt she was supported in her position by eight good and hardworking department heads. She is especially proud that during the last accreditation review no significant deficiencies were reported in any of her departments. She is, however, concerned by the increased competition being presented by Middleboro Community Hospital and feels that Webster Hospital faces an uncertain future, even with the affiliation agreement with OHA. She indicated that the hospital's decision to retain extra staff (and retrain when needed) as it changes its primary orientation away from inpatient services, "made all the difference in the world. Staff became creative problem-solvers because they knew they were not going to lose their jobs."

Wilgus recently headed the management task force that implemented the redesign and expansion of maternity services. For this service, she earned an official commendation from the medical staff. She currently heads the CQI team specifically focusing on clinical and administrative strategies to shorten the length of inpatient hospital stay by diagnosis-related group (DRG). For her past work with this task force, she received a special recognition from the board on the recommendation of Masterman. Masterman recently reminded Wilgus that her recommendations concerning occupational and speech therapy were due on her desk by the end of next month.

Vice President for Clinical Services

Helen Voss, RN, was hired six months ago to fill the vacancy caused by the retirement of Arlene Old, RN. Prior to coming to Webster Hospital, Voss had held numerous nursing positions at Middleboro Community Hospital including being associate director of nursing. She is the first senior employee in 12 years to switch employment between these two hospitals. She is a graduate of the Middleboro Community Hospital School of Nursing and holds an undergraduate degree and master's degree in nursing from State University. She has been very active in the state nursing association. It is noteworthy that she was the unanimous selection of the committee formed to interview all candidates for this position. Voss reports to the president and had responsibility for the following departments:

◆ Clinical education

◆ Pediatrics

◆ Intensive care

◆ Medical surgical unit I

◆ Medical surgical unit II

◆ Medical surgical unit III

◆ Emergency and outpatient departments

◆ Staff development

When interviewed, Voss was careful with her remarks concerning Middleboro Community Hospital and was still unsure concerning the real issues at Webster Hospital. She did say that she was impressed by the high clinical competence of the nursing staff and, unlike Middleboro Community Hospital, was surprised to find that nurse turnover was not a big issue at Webster Hospital. She also indicated that she did not feel threatened by rumors of union activity at Middleboro Community Hospital and did not feel that Webster nurses would follow the lead of the nurses at Middleboro Community Hospital.

Voss cited three factors that convinced her to accept this position. First, the position would not require moving away from Middleboro. Second, she was impressed by the professional relationships between physicians and nurses at Webster Hospital. "Although there is no formal joint practice program, most aspects of joint practice characterize the nurse–physician relationship." Webster Hospital has maintained a high nurse/patient ratio and is continuing to make progress in achieving an all-RN nursing staff. Third, she felt Webster Hospital offered the community a special type of care: "It really cares for its patients, employees, and every member of the Webster family."

When asked specific questions, Voss also opined that the new maternity service in the hospital was state-of-the-art and the basis for the increase in maternity services and births. She also strongly advocated for the hospital continuing to recruit new family practice physicians and develop as many collaborative relationships with physicians as possible.

Director of Marketing

David Story was hired seven years ago in this (then) newly created position. Prior to his appointment he was deputy director of marketing for a durable medical equipment firm in the state capital. He holds an undergraduate degree in liberal arts and a master of health and hospital administration from an eastern university. His family has been especially prominent in Middleboro for many generations. He is a member of ACHE. Initially, when he was hired, he devoted almost all of his time to recruiting physicians. As a result, Story is on a first-name basis with virtually all the physicians on the active medical staff. During his tenure at Webster Hospital he successfully secured the Certificate of Need for a CT scanner and was responsible for all phases of the CT scanner project completed a number of years ago. Prior to the formal affiliation with OHA, he and Swisher negotiated a long-term financial loan with OMC to finance this project. He is currently working with Voss and the medical staff to examine the feasibility of a women's healthcare center at Webster Hospital. He also serves as the director of the physician–hospital organization (PHO) created to facilitate joint ventures between the hospital and members of the medical staff.

When interviewed, Story emphasized the numerous opportunities and threats faced by the hospital. His charge from Masterman—framed on his office wall—is "to work to ensure the survival of Webster Hospital over the long term and help us all develop a true strategic plan." He indicated that Webster Hospital seems well positioned for the future. "We need to continue to build our market share based on serving communities other than just Middleboro. We might need to formally consider a medical office building and even a nursing home on our campus as we evolve into a full-service medical corporation designed to meet the public's needs."

It is interesting to note that Story is proud that he and Swisher are the only two senior managers invited by Masterman to all board meetings.

Management Intern

This advisory staff position to the president is currently held by Mary Hyde. Hyde recently earned a graduate degree in business and hospital administration from a southern university and has been employed by the hospital for seven months as part of the 24-month postgraduate fellowship program recognized by ACHE. Under the terms of this fellowship, the hospital has made no long-term employment commitment to her.

The daughter of an osteopathic physician and holder of an undergraduate degree in psychology, she was a unit manager at a large medical center before entering graduate school. Currently, she provides staff support to various hospital committees and is responsible for the Employee of the Month and Year program. She has completed her administrative rotation and is responsible for a project to upgrade the hospital's guest relations program and data system. Beginning next week she will be providing special assistance to Swisher in human resources administration. Her career interests involve hospital operations. She is a member of ACHE.

MEDICAL STAFF AND MEDICAL RESOURCES

Webster Hospital has 69 osteopathic physicians (DOs) on the active medical staff (see the following chart). All physicians are graduates of osteopathic schools of medicine and have completed internships and residencies in their respective areas of expertise. All physicians added to the active (and consulting) medical staff must be board certified unless this requirement is formally waived by the medical staff's executive committee.

Department	Active	Consulting	Total
Anesthesiology	8	0	8
Emergency medicine	8	4	12
Pathology and radiology	6	6	12
Medicine	36	12	48
Surgery	11	19	30
Total	69	41	110

All physicians on the consulting staff are required to maintain active status on the medical staff of OMC in Capital City or another accredited hospital.

Anesthesiology

The hospital maintains a contractual relationship with DO Anesthesiology Associates PA of Capital City. Four anesthesiologists and four nurse anesthetists are assigned to Webster Hospital. Others are assigned as needed. This professional association also provides support to OMC and most of the other OHA-affiliated hospitals.

Emergency Medicine

The hospital maintains a contractual relationship with DO Emergency and Occupational Health Associates PA of Capital City. Eight physicians are assigned on a permanent basis with other physicians who are brought in as needed. This professional association also provides support to OMC and most of the other OHA-affiliated hospitals.

Pathology and Radiology

The hospital maintains a contractual relationship with DO Pathology Services PA in Capital City. This group has assigned two physicians to provide pathology services. If needed, other pathologists are brought in from Capital City or the procedure is done at OMC. This professional association also provides support to OMC and most of the other OHA-affiliated hospitals.

The hospital also maintains a contractual relationship with DO Radiology Services PA in Capital City. This group has assigned four radiologists to the hospital and provides other services as needed. It should be noted that this group maintains an active computer link between its main and all primary service locations. Using this link, radiologists are able to read and interpret (computer) images and dictate reports. This professional association also provides support to OMC and most of the other OHA-affiliated hospitals.

Department of Medicine

This department includes physicians in private practice. Specialties include general and family practice, internal medicine, pediatrics, cardiology, and ENT. Beginning in 2010 Webster Health System, Inc., began acquiring primary care practices. It now owns 13 medical practices.

Department of Surgery

This department also includes physicians in private practice. Specialties include general surgery, OB/GYN, and orthopedic surgery. Beginning in 2010 Webster Health System, Inc., began acquiring surgical practices. It now owns seven surgical practices.

Medical Staff Organization

Dr. Philip Werner (department of medicine) is president of the medical staff, a position he has held for the last three years. The president is elected every two years and provided a small stipend by the hospital. Meagan Lincoln (pathology) is currently vice-chairman. Dr. Charles Blade (department of surgery) is secretary. Standing committees of the medical staff include the following:

- Utilization review and quality assurance
- Medical records
- Credentials
- Tissue
- Pharmacy and therapeutics
- Executive

The executive committee is composed of the chair of each standing committee as well as the chair of each department and meets monthly or as needed. Other committees also meet monthly. The entire medical staff meets quarterly. The medical staff votes on recredentialing at the annual meeting.

Dr. Werner and selected members of the medical staff were interviewed. Dr. Werner indicated that relations within the medical staff seemed "very professional." He also stated, "Collaboratively, the hospital has helped the medical staff to expand with young, well trained primary care physicians" and "build appropriate referral bridges to OMC." He indicated that some of the older physicians seemed somewhat uncomfortable with the speed but not the substance of many of the recent changes. "Physicians feel included in all phases of this hospital, including its strategic planning." He also shared that being president of the medical staff was becoming "like a full-time job" and that without the stipend provided by the hospital he would be unable to meet many of the expectations.

According to Dr. Werner, the hospital's priorities should include continuing to build up its primary care network, even if this meant building offices and hiring physicians. He felt an immediate priority of Webster Health System, Inc., should be increased ownership of medical practices, medical practice management, and the associated information systems needed to support the business and clinical practice of medicine. He also indicated that medically, the hospital needed to establish a much stronger presence in some of the communities outside Middleboro but said that maintaining any strong presence in Jasper—given the new road—may not be possible or desirable. He also stated, "I'm very impressed with how the hospital has implemented the electronic health record and has had success with meaningful use. I believe we are a model within the OHA system."

Other physicians seemed to agree with Dr. Werner. Dr. Irving Lasker, a member of the medical staff for 32 years, indicated that he was going to retire shortly and hoped that the hospital would continue its expansion. He said the closing of inpatient beds after years of expansion "felt strange, but clearly was the right thing to do." He also stated that the relationship he had with many nurses at Webster Hospital helped him practice high-quality, cost-effective medicine. "The ongoing studies for appropriate ways to shorten lengths of stay are one example of how this hospital has faced up to the challenges and responded appropriately."

Dr. Isaac Kelly, also a long-time member of the medical staff, indicated that he thought that the hospital needed to continue expanding its outpatient services and provide community outreach services to high-risk individuals, especially in the rural area to the north. He also said the medical staff fully supported the acquisition of select medical practices by Webster Hospital and OHA. He indicated that this model removed the burden of managing the practice yet maintained the practice and provided direct access to the hospital's new electronic health record system.

Dr. Alan Able, the newest member of the medical staff, indicated that he saw great possibilities with the existing PHO, strongly supported the continued recruitment of family practice physicians from OMC (like himself), and appreciated the support provided by the hospital to start a thriving practice. "Although we might be located in a rural area, I do not feel isolated. I still have a good relationship with many of the faculty who trained me in medical school at OMC." He also felt that Masterman would be hard to replace.

Dr. Morris Heart was the only physician who offered any critical comments. He was concerned that Webster Hospital has become a medical outpost for OMC. "I am most concerned that OMC physicians—such as Dr. Lincoln—hold leadership positions on our medical staff. Our medical staff has lost the ability to chart its own course. " Dr. Heart's perspective is shared by a small number of other physicians. However, each realizes that if these OMC-contracted physicians were ineligible for these types of positions, even more duties would need to be shared by the physicians in the departments of medicine and surgery. Dr. Heart, however, has remained focused on this issue and has recently written to each physician in these two departments asking that they discuss this issue at their next departmental meeting.

Currently the hospital does not employ hospitalists. As stated by Dr. Werner, "We take care of our own. Maybe someday we will need assistance with inpatient care, but not today." At the same time Dr. Werner has been working on a proposal and contract with OHA for 24-hour hospitalist coverage on weekends. The hospital has taken no position on using hospitalists.

The board of trustees, based on Masterman's recommendation, has recently contracted with a national consulting firm to consider this medical staff issue. The medical staff took no position on the contract, but individual members did suggest that it was inevitable as "we move to more formal medical specialties."

BEHAVIORAL HEALTH

The board of OHAHS has recently recommended that OHA develop one or more dedicated units in its affiliated hospitals that specialize in the treatment of drug and alcohol addiction and that once these units are established, "at least one of the hospitals also develop a comprehensive inpatient psychiatric facility to serve the entire OHA system." Webster Hospital has a long-standing agreement with the Middleboro Counseling Center for inpatient emergency psychiatric services, including suicide watch. Under this agreement, an emergency psychiatric admission is limited to 48 hours before the patient must be transferred and the total number of inpatient days is capped at 100 per year. This report indicates that Webster Hospital is one of the current affiliates that should be considered for a dedicated behavioral health (e.g., drug and alcohol) unit or side-by-side facility and has furnished Webster Hospital the following information.

Note that OHAHS has previously determined that a significant number of patients from Webster Hospital's service area seek drug and alcohol treatment services in Capital City. OHAHS also estimates that Webster, because of its cost structure, may be able to provide a competitive plan for patients and corporations in Capital City and University Town.

Story, working with OHA, has estimated that a mature program—assuming aggressive advertising and promotion—should be able to serve up to 85 percent of the market within 40 miles and 40 percent of the market located between 41 and 80 miles of the facility.

DRUG AND ALCOHOL SERVICE COST ESTIMATES

- Physical facilities: Must be physically isolated in the hospital with restricted access. It is preferable that drug and alcohol patients do not share the same room.
- Renovation costs of existing space: Estimated at $150 per square foot.
- New construction costs: Estimated at $325 per square foot exclusive of land purchase and site preparation (if any).

Design Consideration	Square-Foot Requirement	Comment
Each semiprivate room	400	
Reception area	1,600	
Counseling office	400	1 needed for every 10 beds
Commons, hallways	2,500	Per every 20 beds
General purpose room	1,600	Minimum of 1; 1 additional for each 40 beds

Estimated Utilization Factors Covering Drug and Alcohol Services: Community Hospital–Based Programs

A drug and alcohol program is typically offered in three phases:

Phase I   Inpatient detoxification and medical examination

Phase II   Inpatient rehabilitation/counseling/family therapy

Phase III Hospital-sponsored outpatient counseling

Further study is needed to define the program's actual configuration. Recidivism rates for 7-, 14-, and 21-day inpatient program (Phase II) need to be considered.

(continued)

(continued from previous page)

Annual Admission Rate per 1,000 (Age 25 and Older)

Alcohol	1.9
Drug	0.7

Drug and Alcohol Utilization Factors by Gender and Age, Community Hospital–Based Programs (Age 25 and Older)

Program	Gender	Average Age	Percent
Alcohol	Male	42.4	78
	Female	37.6	22
Drug	Male	29.6	70
	Female	32.2	30

Purchasing estimates for equipment purchased through OHA

Hospital bed	$12,500
Other room furnishing per bed	5,650
Counseling office furniture	1,600
Reception-area furniture	2,900
General purpose furniture (TV plus other)	6,000

Staffing for a program must include a designated medical director to manage Phase I and oversee as needed Phase II. The inpatient service (e.g., Phase II) needs appropriately trained nurses and certified counselors. Phase III also needs certified counselors.

Insurance Information

Blue Cross and Blue Shield, area HMOs, and managed care plans pay charges based on a "not to exceed" dollar level per admission of $12,500, with the stipulation that no eligible enrollees can use this benefit more than twice.

Medicare (Part A) pays charges minus 10 percent. Commercial insurance pays $1,000 per patient day, with a lifetime maximum of $20,000. Medicaid pays $210 per inpatient day for Phase I; Medicaid does not reimburse other services.

Webster Hospital has agreed to take this information under advisement and report back to OHA in 60 days whether it is interested in establishing a dedicated drug and alcohol unit or donating land adjacent to the hospital for a joint project (and new facility) with OMC. It should be noted that OHA plans to establish two or three of these behavioral units in or adjacent to its affiliated hospitals. OHA has previously determined that its first psychiatric facility should be located outside Capital City but within a 150-mile radius of Capital City. When asked, OHA said it has not ruled out the possibility of developing this service line using OHAV, Inc.

Other Information

OHA is considering a program to brand all affiliated hospitals on quality and privacy. It has asked each of its affiliated hospitals to indicate its potential bed needs for 2015 and beyond and undertake a study to determine the financial ramifications of making all inpatient medical–surgical beds private, in contrast to semiprivate. It has estimated that existing semiprivate rooms could be modified into private rooms for $425,000 per room, and new private rooms (a minimum of 10) could be added for approximately $1 million per bed. (Values expressed in 2014 dollars.) OHA has indicated that the analysis should assume a 20-year straight-line depreciation approach and no salvage values. OHA has indicated that it can commit to up to 100 percent financing at an annual interest rate not to exceed 4 percent.

It is common knowledge that Jennifer Kip and Alan Simpson, members of the Jasper City Council, have approached the governor about a plan for a hospital in Jasper. According to Kip, "Residents in Jasper need access to a hospital, especially an emergency department; too many of our residents have to travel too many miles when they most need these types of services." The governor has met with them and recommended that they work with the State Commissioner of Health and Welfare to determine whether a small hospital in Jasper is a viable venture. The governor has promised his support to ensure that the residents "of this growing community have access to the type of health service services they need and can support." Kip and Simpson have told the press that they will ask the Jasper City Council to authorize the retention of a consulting firm to study this issue. This issue was discussed when the hospital's medical staff last met with Masterman.

Eric Martin, a member of the hospital's board, has asked Masterman to consider what Webster should do given that Physician Care Services, Inc. (PCS) is (apparently) for sale. According to Martin, PCS has provided his company occupational health services for the past two years—"lowering our worker comp costs and occupational health costs at least 15 percent in the process"—and is one of the reasons that his company is no longer considering relocating out of the area.

At the last board meeting, Daniel Will, the board chairman, asked each board member to come to the next meeting prepared to help prepare the profile of "the next president for this hospital," a profile to be furnished to national recruiting firms in anticipation of Masterman's retirement. He specifically asked each board member to express an opinion as to whether the president should or should not have a clinical background. He indicated that the following issues must be addressed:

◆ Concerning the Patient Protection and Affordable Care Act and accountable care organizations, detailed plans need to be developed and implemented.

◆ Within the next three to five years, how should the hospital recruit physicians? Should recruitment emphasize primary care or specialty care? Does Webster Hospital need to recruit to replace specific physicians and surgeons? How many physicians and surgeons are located where should the hospital be considering?

◆ The potential need to hire a chief information officer and establish an in-house information systems staff to support operations and hospital-owned medical practices. What is the future of Webster Hospital's existing consulting and service contracts used to address this need?

◆ The need and demand for new surgical technologies. Which new technologies should Webster Hospital prioritize?

◆ Should the hospital establish a hospital outpatient clinic in the northern rural area? Where should or could this clinic be located? What services should be provided? What are the associated costs and benefits?

◆ What are the ramifications of a (rumored) 15 to 20 percent increase in OHA membership costs?

◆ Can the hospital continue its ten-year plan to earn LEED (Leadership in Energy and Environmental Design) certification?

The recent release of the IRS Form 990 shows that the 2014 salaries for the ten highest-paid Webster Hospital employees are:

Name	Position	2014 Salary
Janice Masterman	President and CEO	$540,000
Steve Swisher	CFO	283,000
Helen Voss, RN	VP, clinical services	198,500
Mary Help, RN	Associate VP, clinical services	132,040
Carla Fox	Associate VP, administrative services/director of medical records	110,340
Ellen Wilgus	VP, professional services	105,370
David Story	Director of marketing	104,220
Cheryl Watkins	Associate VP, finance	95,230
David Crow	Laboratory director	94,500
Alex Ham	Pharmacy director	93,440

Compensation also includes benefits, which are 40 percent above salary. For every $1,000 in salary, total compensation includes an additional $400 for benefits. Emergency services, radiology, pathology and anesthesiology are provided by contract with specific private corporations. The hospital does not directly employ any physicians in these specialties.

Note that Webster Health System, Inc., owns and operates medical practices in support of the mission and goals of Webster Hospital.

Additional information regarding Webster Hospital's staffing, utilization, financial status, payer mix, and patient demographics may be found in the following tables.

TABLE 4.1
Webster Hospital
Medical Staff
Information, 2014

Name	Office	Age	Specialty	Patients	Discharges
Department of Medicine—Active Staff					
General and Family Practice					
A. Able	1	29	Family Practice*	504	115
A. Adelson	1	33	Family Practice*	601	125
A. Downs	1	34	Family Practice*	678	152
B. Dawes	1	34	Family Practice*	590	146
B. Lamb	1	37	Family Practice*	603	149
C. Franklin	2	48	Family Practice	323	66
C. Newton	2	44	Family Practice	476	96
D. Dodger	3	37	Family Practice*	415	91
E. Best	3	35	Family Practice*	340	84
E. Devishson	3	31	Family Practice*	186	43
E. Doogle	3	36	Family Practice*	357	82
F. Walczek	5	38	Family Practice	300	64
F. Evans	4	39	Family Practice	197	45
G. Liu	6	29	Family Practice	287	50
H. Megg	7	36	Family Practice	454	100
J. Child	4	43	Family Practice	244	55
J. Kim	4	32	Family Practice	456	91
J. Lopez	1	40	Family Practice	478	103
K. Blood	1	50	Family Practice	534	109
K. Justin	2	57	Family Practice	539	114
M. Heart	1	43	Family Practice	478	101
B. Easter	1	68	General Practice	547	102
C. Fisher	2	60	General Practice	416	92
D. Hamilton	2	55	General Practice	345	77
I. Kelly	8	69	General Practice	38	7
I. Lasker	8	68	General Practice	135	24

(continued)

Name	Office	Age	Specialty	Patients	Discharges
Internal Medicine: General					
J. Morgan	1	35	Internal Medicine	590	121
K. Organs	1	54	Internal Medicine	398	86
Pediatrics					
D. White	1	34	Pediatrics*	162	45
H. Wall	1	37	Pediatrics*	45	18
N. Green	1	35	Pediatrics*	80	28
X. Hirsh	1	39	Pediatrics*	40	15
Cardiology					
W. Snipes	3	45	Cardiology	546	105
Other: Medicine					
A. Zook	1	57	Endocrinology	129	24
J. Hogan	1	50	ENT	365	70
P. Taff	1	43	ENT	356	66
Department of Medicine—Consulting Staff					
J. Washington	3	43	Internal Medicine	65	10
C. Eisenhower	9	50	Cardiology	243	41
S. Truman	9	43	Rheumatology	334	62
L. Coolidge	3	44	ENT	143	31
W. G. Chan	3	37	Pediatrics	132	25
W. Tafy	9	57	Oncology	356	50
V. Kennedy	3	64	ENT	140	26
T. Johnson	9	47	Cardiology	176	32
C. Nixon	9	54	Internal Medicine	160	24
M. Polk	3	40	OB/GYN	112	20
S. Warren	9	50	Pulmonary Medicine	655	113

TABLE 4.1

Webster Hospital Medical Staff Information, 2014 (continued)

(continued)

Name	Office	Age	Specialty	Patients	Discharges
T. Werner	9	53	Pulmonary Medicine	503	90
Others	9			168	32
Department of Surgery					
General and Orthopedic					
S. Saw	1	31	General*	759	155
C. Blade	1	50	General*	671	142
R. Runner	1	37	Orthopedic	766	155
D. Dolittle	1	46	Orthopedic	792	164
Other					
D. Felix	1	47	Urology	403	77
OB/GYN					
B. Shaw	1	40	OB/GYN*	415	90
D. Kirby	1	43	OB/GYN	403	92
E. Munson	1	44	OB/GYN*	403	95
F. Zebra	1	41	OB/GYN*	602	129
G. Martinez	1	47	OB/GYN*	621	143
M. Lewis	1	49	OB/GYN*	678	137
Surgery—Consulting Staff					
M. Merrill	9	47	General	48	8
W. Pierce	9	51	General	153	27
F. Stevensen	3	61	General	100	19
J. Tyler	3	63	General	140	26
P. Miller	3	68	General	45	7
J. McKinley	3	65	General	32	5
M. Dawes	10	56	General	116	20
S. Strimpf	10	54	General	124	22

(continued)

Name	Office	Age	Specialty	Patients	Discharges
S. Skier	9	54	Orthopedic	216	41
W. Hockey	9	47	Orthopedic	106	20
S. Fremont	9	45	Orthopedic	95	18
M. Fremont	9	45	Orthopedic	96	16
D. Davids	9	50	Orthopedic	54	10
K. Nioxon	9	63	Orthopedic	20	3
G. Grant	9	50	Orthopedic	22	4
L. Goldwater	3	44	Orthopedic	20	3
W. Miller	3	47	Orthopedic	27	5
D. Garfield	9	43	Thoracic	59	9
K. McGovern	9	53	Thoracic	105	16
D. Chest	9	50	Thoracic	145	20
Department of Pathology and Radiology—Active Staff					
J. Ericksen	1	48	Radiology		
H. Holland	1	62	Radiology		
W. Jippel	1	46	Radiology		
D. Yip	1	43	Pathology		
M. Stern	1	44	Pathology		
M. Lincoln	1	34	Pathology		
Department of Pathology and Radiology—Consulting Staff					
M. Currie	9	58	Radiology		
D. Douglas	9	43	Radiology		
W. Lewis	9	40	Radiology		
D. Slide	9	55	Pathology		
F. Fillerautz	9	44	Pathology		
G. Gathews	9	47	Pathology		

TABLE 4.1

Webster Hospital Medical Staff Information, 2014 (continued)

(continued)

TABLE 4.1

Webster Hospital
Medical Staff
Information, 2014
(continued)

Name	Office	Age	Specialty	Patients	Discharges
Department of Anesthesiology—Active Staff					
N. Needle	1	38	Anesthesiology		
S. Westerman	1	42	Anesthesiology		
N. Chamerblin	1	44	Anesthesiology		
S. Pak	1	54	Anesthesiology		
D. Sleep	9	61	Anesthesiology		
M. Halo	9	50	Anesthesiology		
J. Jones	9	46	Anesthesiology		
D. Dinckens	9	41	Anesthesiology		
Department of Emergency Medicine—Active Staff					
E. Abelson	1	44	Emergency		
M. Gasp	1	51	Emergency		
I. Hurt	1	42	Emergency		
A. Lincoln	1	34	Emergency		
H. Calson	1	40	Emergency		
W. Hiller	1	47	Emergency		
S. Sams	1	45	Emergency		
G. Bodansky	1	50	Emergency		
Department of Emergency Medicine—Consulting Staff					
J. Whitney	9	47	Emergency		
J. Sallowash	9	51	Emergency		
R. Ritco	9	41	Emergency		
TBD	9		Emergency		

NOTES

* = Medical practice owned by Webster Health System, Inc.

Office Location: 1=Middleboro; 2=Mifflenville; 3=Jasper; 4=Harris City; 5=Statesville; 6 = Carterville; 7 = Boalsburg; 8=Minortown; 9=Capital City; 10=Other.

(This table can also be found online at ache.org/books/Middleboro.)

Hospital Service	2014	2013	2012	2011	2010	2009	2008
Pediatrics							
Beds	2	2	3	4	4	4	6
Patient days	450	645	706	804	903	998	1,212
Occupancy	61.6%	88.4%	64.5%	55.1%	61.8%	68.4%	55.3%
Maternity							
Beds	20	20	14	14	14	11	10
Patient days	5,470	4,956	4,106	3,845	3,455	2,840	2,740
Occupancy	74.9%	67.9%	80.4%	75.2%	67.6%	70.7%	75.1%
Medical Surgical I							
Beds	20	20	22	20	20	18	20
Patient days	5,270	6,047	6,070	5,578	6,129	4,996	5,582
Occupancy	72.2%	82.8%	75.6%	76.4%	84.0%	76.0%	76.5%
Medical Surgical II							
Beds	20	20	23	21	21	24	21
Patient days	5,442	5,163	5,890	5,830	5,770	6,556	5,979
Occupancy	74.5%	70.7%	70.2%	76.1%	75.3%	74.8%	78.0%
Medical Surgical III							
Beds	20	20	20	20	20	21	20
Patient days	5,067	6,089	5,378	5,503	5,586	5,767	5,830
Occupancy	69.4%	83.4%	73.7%	75.4%	76.5%	75.2%	79.9%
Orthopedic							
Beds	0	0	4	7	8	12	13
Patient days	0	0	955	1845	2140	3324	3824
Occupancy	0.0%	0.0%	65.4%	72.2%	73.3%	75.9%	80.6%
ICU							
Beds	13	13	12	12	11	10	10
Patient days	2,956	2,802	2,655	2,282	1,981	1,810	1,567
Occupancy	62.3%	59.1%	60.6%	52.1%	49.3%	49.6%	42.9%
Total Hospital							
Beds	95	95	98	98	98	100	100
Patient days	24,655	25,702	25,760	25,687	25,964	26,291	26,734
Occupancy	71.1%	74.1%	72.0%	71.8%	72.6%	72.0%	73.2%

TABLE 4.2
Hospital Inpatient Occupancy by Service, 2008–2014

(This table can also be found online at ache.org/books/Middleboro.)

TABLE 4.3

Detailed Utilization
Statistics, 2014 and
2013

2014	Discharges	Patient Days	Inpatient Surgery	Outpatient Surgery	Births	ED Visits	ED Admits	OPV
January	412	2,133	103	407	124	1,798	215	6,962
February	387	1,894	104	367	105	1,676	200	6,072
March	507	2,060	112	427	124	1,803	234	7,245
April	499	1,978	107	419	136	1,830	220	7,520
May	409	2,178	105	434	121	1,795	218	7,029
June	389	2,056	101	495	123	1,798	212	6,998
July	353	2,157	102	412	115	1,823	219	7,126
August	375	1,867	90	390	127	1,880	230	6,349
September	435	2,245	114	408	139	1,748	200	7,836
October	423	1,956	116	417	136	1,850	213	7,354
November	494	2,059	103	426	134	1,880	223	6,926
December	412	2,072	99	403	126	1,675	200	6,559
Total	**5,095**	**24,655**	**1,256**	**5,005**	**1,510**	**21,556**	**2,584**	**83,976**
2013								
January	312	2,056	117	405	121	1,662	200	6,956
February	433	1,928	104	401	108	1,640	196	5,728
March	446	2,186	116	417	110	1,658	199	6,689
April	400	2,001	137	423	124	1,640	190	7,387
May	445	1,978	132	422	108	1,720	201	7,704
June	412	1,905	113	395	118	1,710	200	7,005
July	408	2,156	105	366	114	1,720	206	6,129
August	407	2,169	95	382	113	1,820	212	5,946
September	405	2,190	134	410	118	1,748	209	7,558
October	434	2,101	120	412	137	1,743	214	7,054
November	490	2,067	116	418	122	1,734	204	7,067
December	541	2,265	109	419	106	1,656	188	6,126
Total	**5,133**	**25,002**	**1,398**	**4,870**	**1,399**	**20,451**	**2,419**	**81,349**

NOTES:
ED Visits = Total emergency department visits
ED Admits = ED visits that led to an inpatient admission
OPV = Outpatient visits, excludes ED visits

(This table can also be found online at ache.org/books/Middleboro.)

Revenue	2014	2013	2012
Patient services revenue—total	**290,117,301**	**288,362,045**	**287,223,124**
Inpatient	105,718,744	109,577,577	116,919,656
Outpatient	184,398,557	178,784,468	170,303,468
Allowances and uncollectables—inpatient	50,744,997	53,667,342	55,341,870
Allowances and uncollectables—outpatient	103,017,173	102,048,162	99,758,617
Total	153,762,170	155,715,504	155,100,487
Net service revenue	**136,355,131**	**132,646,541**	**132,122,637**
Other operating revenue	108,330	88,453	72,290
Total operating revenue	**136,463,461**	**132,734,994**	**132,194,927**
Expenses			
Operating expense			
Patient care services	43,245,232	40,384,554	38,345,292
Other professional services	30,898,223	30,556,393	30,573,990
General services	24,836,292	22,405,239	23,450,202
Fiscal and admin services	24,638,272	24,003,292	24,595,281
Interest	1,865,693	1,813,907	1,936,889
Depreciation	5,320,108	5,891,202	5,412,404
Community education and outreach	251,799	299,874	225,665
Total operating expenses	**131,055,619**	**125,354,461**	**124,539,723**
Net income from operation	**5,407,842**	**7,380,533**	**7,655,204**
Nonoperating revenue			
Unrestricted gifts and bequests	198,233	147,841	111,343
Income from investments	3,059,282	3,017,334	3,005,264
Miscellaneous nonpatient revenue	1,118,332	1,000,785	957,223
Total	**4,375,847**	**3,165,175**	**3,116,607**
Nonoperating expenses	**2,554,293**	**2,007,343**	**3,402,348**
Net nonoperating income	**1,821,554**	**1,157,832**	**(285,741)**
Profit (loss)	**7,229,396**	**8,538,365**	**10,771,811**

TABLE 4.4

Statement of Revenue and Expense for Calendar Years Ending December 31 ($)

(This table can also be found online at ache.org/books/Middleboro.)

TABLE 4.5

Balance Sheet as of December 31 ($)

	2014	2013	2012
Current assets			
Cash	3,005,494	2,324,303	2,439,495
Short-term investments	3,035,445	2,224,383	893,247
Accounts receivable—gross	33,458,282	34,292,554	36,595,230
Allowances for uncollectables	18,563,987	19,393,554	19,937,554
Accounts receivable—net	14,894,295	14,899,000	16,657,676
Due from third-party payers	607,255	349,228	103,450
Inventories	4,866,345	4,995,395	5,394,129
Prepaid expenses	153,702	176,872	162,508
Total current assets	**26,562,536**	**24,969,181**	**25,650,505**
Noncurrent assets			
Property, plant, and equipment—gross	107,353,474	104,393,556	100,384,345
Less accumulated depreciation	67,334,262	62,014,154	56,122,952
Property, plant, and equipment—net	40,019,212	42,379,402	44,261,393
Other investments	14,997,675	14,349,292	8,530,204
Total assets	**81,579,423**	**81,697,875**	**78,442,102**
Current liabilities			
Accounts payable	5,334,675	5,539,564	5,420,787
Accrued salaries and wages	767,056	828,349	792,414
Accrued interest	107,342	72,204	70,245
Other accrued expenses	279,474	261,584	270,654
Due to third-party vendors	705,613	702,461	582,491
Long-term debt due within one year	2,158,337	1,345,965	945,229
Total current liabilities	**9,352,497**	**8,750,127**	**8,081,820**
Long-term debt	20,456,294	28,500,704	34,282,450
Total liabilities	**29,808,791**	**37,250,831**	**42,364,270**
Net assets			
Restricted	6,128,484	6,034,292	6,203,445
Unrestricted	45,642,148	38,506,944	29,799,426
Total net assets	**51,770,632**	**44,541,236**	**36,002,871**

(This table can also be found online at ache.org/books/Middleboro.)

DRG Name	Number of Discharges					
	2014	2013	2012	2011	2010	2009
Normal newborn[1]	1,389	1,287	1,147	1,066	1,074	1,032
Vaginal delivery, no complications	1,022	945	821	745	756	801
Caesarean section	414	377	346	312	328	301
Medical back problems	412	487	523	480	532	742
Chest pain	284	248	287	317	289	325
Simple pneumonia and pleurisy	151	178	192	168	156	147
Coronary atherosclerosis	147	148	139	196	156	175
Other digestive system diagnoses	138	142	154	138	129	178
Major joint or reattachment of lower extremity	99	90	78	89	95	90
Cholecystectomy	76	83	57	67	72	69
Total top ten, excluding births	2,743	2,698	2,597	2,512	2,513	2,828
Total hospital discharges	5,095	5,326	5,362	5,412	5,769	5,790
Percent top ten, excluding births	53.84%	50.66%	48.43%	46.42%	43.56%	48.84%

TABLE 4.6
Top Ten DRGs, 2009–2014

1. Counted as births, not discharges.

TABLE 4.7
Patient Days by Type and Type of Payer, 2014

Type of Patient Day	Total Patient Days	Medicare	Medicaid	BC HMO	BC PPO	BC Indemnity	Swift	CS PPO	Comm PPO	Comm Indemnity	Other	Self-Pay
Medical	27.1%	10.3%	3.9%	0.0%	0.0%	5.9%	0.0%	1.5%	0.0%	4.2%	0.2%	1.1%
Surgical												
Nonorthopedic	13.4%	5.4%	2.2%	0.2%	0.3%	1.1%	0.0%	0.3%	0.0%	3.0%	0.3%	0.6%
Orthopedic	6.7%	2.3%	1.1%	0.2%	0.1%	1.3%	0.0%	0.0%	0.0%	1.1%	0.1%	0.5%
OB	22.8%	0.0%	2.7%	1.1%	6.7%	3.0%	0.0%	0.8%	0.0%	4.2%	0.5%	3.8%
Newborn	11.0%	0.0%	2.3%	0.9%	1.4%	3.0%	0.0%	0.2%	0.0%	2.4%	0.3%	0.5%
Other pediatric	1.8%	0.0%	1.1%	0.3%	0.0%	0.1%	0.0%	0.1%	0.0%	0.0%	0.0%	0.2%
ICU/CCU	12.0%	5.4%	0.7%	0.2%	0.2%	2.4%	0.0%	0.3%	0.0%	1.6%	0.5%	0.7%
Psychological	4.2%	2.0%	0.2%	0.0%	0.0%	0.0%	0.0%	0.0%	0.0%	0.0%	0.0%	2.0%
Substance abuse												
Detox	0.0%	0.0%	0.0%	0.0%	0.0%	0.0%	0.0%	0.0%	0.0%	0.0%	0.0%	0.0%
Rehab	1.0%	0.5%	0.0%	0.0%	0.0%	0.3%	0.0%	0.0%	0.0%	0.2%	0.0%	0.0%
Total	**100.0%**	**25.9%**	**14.2%**	**2.9%**	**8.7%**	**17.1%**	**0.0%**	**3.2%**	**0.0%**	**16.7%**	**1.9%**	**9.4%**

NOTES
BC = Blue Cross
CS = Central States Good Health Network
Swift = Swift Health Plan
Comm = Commercial

Category	CMS Core Measure	State Benchmark	WH 2014	WH 2013	WH 2012
Timely Heart Attack Care	Average number of minutes before outpatient with chest pain or possible heart attack who needed specialized care was transferred to another hospital	1 hr	n/a	n/a	n/a
Timely Heart Attack Care	Average number of minutes before outpatient with chest pain or possible heart attack got an ECG	8 min	6 min	n/a	n/a
Timely Heart Attack Care	Outpatients with chest pain or possible heart attack who got aspirin within 24 hours of arrival	100%	90%	87%	91%
Timely Heart Attack Care	Heart attack patients given PCI within 90 minutes of arrival	94%	86%	88%	94%
Effective Heart Attack Care	Heart attack patients given aspirin at discharge	100%	100%	99%	100%
Effective Heart Attack Care	Heart attack patients given a prescription for a statin at discharge	97%	97%	98%	98%
Effective Heart Failure Care	Heart failure patients given discharge instructions	92%	93%	92%	93%
Effective Heart Failure Care	Heart failure patients given an evaluation of left ventricular systolic (LVS) function	97%	100%	100%	100%
Effective Heart Failure Care	Heart failure patients given ACE inhibitor or ARB for left ventricular systolic dysfunction (LVSD)	97%	97%	96%	100%
Effective Pneumonia Care	Pneumonia patients whose initial emergency department blood culture was performed prior to the administration of the hospital dose of antibiotics	97%	98%	98%	98%

TABLE 4.8
CMS Core Measures for Webster Hospital (WH), 2012–2014

(continued)

Category	CMS Core Measure	State Benchmark	WH 2014	WH 2013	WH 2012
Effective Pneumonia Care	Pneumonia patients given the most appropriate initial antibiotics	96%	96%	94%	95%
Timely Surgical Care	Outpatients having surgery who got an antibiotic at the right time (within one hour before surgery)	98%	99%	98%	98%
Timely Surgical Care	Surgery patients who were given an antibiotic at the right time (within one hour before surgery) to help prevent infection	98%	98%	98%	98%
Timely Surgical Care	Surgery patients whose preventive antibiotics were stopped at the right time (within 24 hours after surgery)	97%	98%	99%	98%
Timely Surgical Care	Patients who got treatment at the right time (within 24 hours before or after their surgery) to help prevent blood clot after certain types of surgery	97%	96%	98%	98%
Effective Surgical Care	Outpatients having surgery who got the right kind of antibiotic	98%	99%	99%	98%
Effective Surgical Care	Surgery patients who were taking beta blockers before coming to the hospital, who were kept on the beta blockers during the period just before and after the surgery	96%	100%	96%	98%
Effective Surgical Care	Surgery patients who were given the right kind of antibiotic to help prevent infection	98%	100%	97%	96%
Effective Surgical Care	Heart surgery patients whose blood sugar is kept under good control in the days right after surgery	95%	n/a	n/a	n/a

(continued)

Category	CMS Core Measure	State Benchmark	WH 2014	WH 2013	WH 2012
Effective Surgical Care	Surgery patients whose urinary catheters were removed on the first or second day after surgery	94%	96%	96%	96%
Effective Surgical Care	Patients having surgery who were actively warmed in the operating room or whose body temperature was near normal by the end of surgery	100%	100%	100%	100%
Effective Surgical Care	Surgery patients whose doctor ordered treatments to prevent blood clots after certain types of surgeries	98%	99%	98%	99%
Emergency Department (ED) Care	Average (median) time patient spent in the ED before they were admitted to the hospital as an inpatient (minutes)	Being developed	338	n/a	n/a
Emergency Department (ED) Care	Average (median) time patient spent in the ED, after the doctor decided to admit them as an inpatient before leaving the ED for inpatient care (minutes)	Being developed	146	n/a	n/a
Emergency Department (ED) Care	Average time patients spent in the ED before being sent home (minutes)	Being developed	125	n/a	n/a
Emergency Department (ED) Care	Average time patients who came to the ED with broken bones had to wait before receiving pain medication (minutes)	Being developed	35	n/a	n/a
Emergency Department (ED) Care	Percentage of patients who left the ED before being seen	Being developed	3%	n/a	n/a
Emergency Department (ED) Care	Percentage of patients who came to the ED with stroke symptoms who received brain scan results within 45 minutes of arrival	Being developed	n/a	n/a	n/a

TABLE 4.8
CMS Core Measures for Webster Hospital (WH), 2012–2014 (continued)

(continued)

Category	CMS Core Measure	State Benchmark	WH 2014	WH 2013	WH 2012
Preventive Care	Patients assessed and given influenza vaccination	95%	73%	n/a	n/a
Preventive Care	Patients assessed and given pneumonia vaccination	93%	78%	n/a	n/a
Readmission, Complications and Death	Rate of readmission for heart attack	No different from US national rate			
Readmission, Complications and Death	Death rate for heart attack patients	No different from US national rate			
Readmission, Complications and Death	Rate of readmission for heart failure patients	No different from US national rate			
Readmission, Complications and Death	Rate of readmission for pneumonia patients	No different from US national rate			
Readmission, Complications and Death	Death rate for pneumonia patients	Better than US national rate			
Serious Complications and Deaths	Serious complications rate	No different from US national rate			
Hospital Acquired Conditions	Hospital-acquired conditions	Being developed	n/a	n/a	n/a
Healthcare Associated Infections	Central line–associated bloodstream infections	No different from the US national benchmark			
Use of Medical Imaging	Outpatients with low back pain who had an MRI without trying recommended treatments first, such as PT (percent)	32.9%	27%	28%	31%

(continued)

Category	CMS Core Measure	State Benchmark	WH 2014	WH 2013	WH 2012
Use of Medical Imaging	Outpatients who had a follow-up mammogram or ultrasound within 45 days after a screening mammogram (percent)	12.40%	5%	5%	8%
Use of Medical Imaging	Outpatient CT scans of the chest that were "combination" scans (percent)	0.03%	<1%	<1%	<1%
Use of Medical Imaging	Outpatient CT scans of the abdomen that were "combination" scans (percent)	0.07%	<1%	<1%	<1%
Use of Medical Imaging	Outpatients who got cardiac imaging stress tests before low-risk outpatient surgery (percent)	Being developed	6%	6%	7%
Use of Medical Imaging	Outpatients with brain CT scans who got a sinus CT scan at the same time (percent)	Being developed	4%	4%	4%
Patient Survey Results	Patients who reported that their nurses "always" communicated well (percent)	84%	82%	84%	83%
Patient Survey Results	Patients who reported that their doctor "always" communicated well (percent)	80%	84%	84%	77%
Patient Survey Results	Patients who reported they "always" received help as soon as they wanted (percent)	62%	69%	66%	66%
Patient Survey Results	Patients who reported that their pain was "always" well controlled (percent)	75%	72%	71%	71%
Patient Survey Results	Patients who reported that staff "always" explained about medicines before administering them (percent)	69%	64%	64%	62%

TABLE 4.8
CMS Core Measures for Webster Hospital (WH), 2012–2014 (continued)

(continued)

Category	CMS Core Measure	State Benchmark	WH 2014	WH 2013	WH 2012
Patient Survey Results	Patients who reported that their room and bathroom were "always" clean	73%	78%	74%	74%
Patient Survey Results	Patients who reported that the area around their room was "always" quiet at night	73%	55%	53%	51%
Patient Survey Results	Patients at each hospital who reported "yes," they were given information about what to do during their recovery at home.	85%	92%	88%	89%
Patient Survey Results	Patients who gave their hospital a rating of 9 or 10 on a scale from 0 to 10.	68%	71%	72%	70%
Patient Survey Results	Patients who reported "yes," they would definitely recommend the hospital	76%	80%	75%	76%

NOTE: "n/a" means either that the data are not available or that the number of cases is too small for any legitimate conclusion. "Being developed" means that the core measure remains under development and no standard or benchmark has been published.

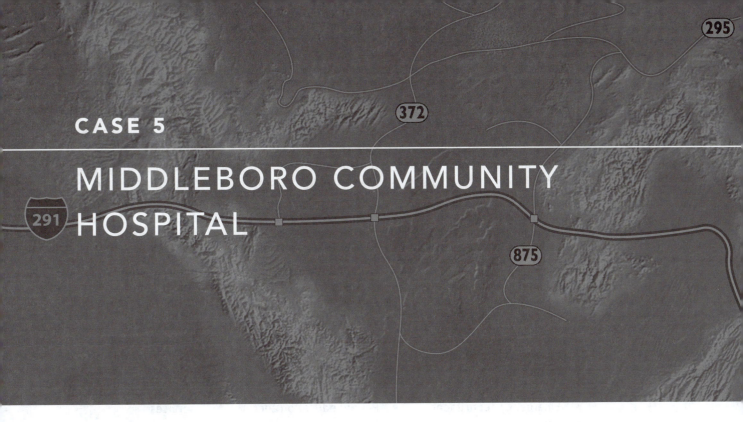

CASE 5

MIDDLEBORO COMMUNITY HOSPITAL

Middleboro Community Hospital (MCH) was founded as a short-term, general acute-care nonprofit hospital in 1890. Originally built with a 40-bed capacity, it has slowly grown to its present 272-bed size and has added a significant number of outpatient services. MCH is licensed by the state, incorporated as a 501(c)3 nonprofit corporation, accredited by The Joint Commission, approved by the American College of Surgeons (cancer program), approved for Blue Cross participation, certified by the US Department of Health and Human Services for participation in Medicare, and accepts Medicaid patients. The Joint Commission recently granted a five-year accreditation based on periodic surveys. Current services, as indicated on the most recent survey by the American Hospital Association, include the following:

- Airborne infection isolation room
- Auxiliary organization
- Bariatric/weight control services
- Birthing room, LDR room, LDRP Room
- Cardiac intensive care
- Cardiac rehabilitation
- Extracorporeal shock wave lithotripter
- Health fair
- Community health education
- Health screening
- Health research
- Hemodialysis
- HIV/AIDS services
- Multislice spiral computed tomography, <64-slice CT
- Multislice spiral computed tomography, 64+ slice CT
- Positron emission tomography
- Positron emission tomography/CT
- Ultrasound

- Adult interventional cardiac catheterization
- Case management
- Chaplaincy/pastoral care
- Chemotherapy
- Children's wellness program
- Community health reporting
- Community health status assessment
- Community health status–based service planning
- Community outreach
- Complementary and alternative medicine
- Emergency department
- Enabling services
- Palliative care program
- Optical colonoscopy
- Endoscopic ultrasound
- Ablation of Barrett's esophagus
- Endoscopic retrograde
- Enrollment assistance services
- Electron beam computed tomography
- Hospital-based outpatient care center services
- Immunization program
- Medical–surgical intensive care services
- Neurological services
- Nutritional programs
- Obstetrics
- Occupational health services
- Oncology services
- Orthopedic services
- Other special care
- Outpatient surgery
- Patient controlled analgesia
- Patient education center
- Physical rehabilitation inpatient services
- Physical rehabilitation outpatient services
- Prosthetic and orthotic services
- CT scanner
- Diagnostic radioisotope facility
- Magnetic resonance imaging
- Image-guided radiation therapy
- Intensity-modulated radiation therapy
- Shaped beam radiation system
- Genetic testing/counseling
- Robotic surgery
- Sleep center
- Social work services
- Sports medicine
- Support groups
- Tobacco treatment/cessation program
- Transportation to health services
- Urgent care center
- Virtual colonoscopy
- Volunteer services department
- Women's health center/services
- Wound management services

HISTORY AND PHYSICAL STRUCTURE

Since its construction, MCH has been a model of hospital engineering and community interest. The hospital replaced three area homes used for the care of the sick. Today, the hospital is a fully air-conditioned, five-floor brick facility on a 68-acre campus. Ample parking is provided. Over the years increasing service demands required additions to the original structure. Each time these additions were built, existing facilities were modernized. Fund-raising campaigns raised the majority of resources for additions completed in 1924 and 1946. Federal Hill-Burton funds were used to partially finance the 1952 and 1966 additions. The 2002 building program relied on retained earnings, community philanthropy, and long-term borrowing.

In 1919, this hospital founded a school of nursing to train area personnel. This three-year diploma school was one of the largest in the state and trained many of the nurses currently working at the hospital. In 1985 however, the increasing costs of the school, the declining interest of local residents, and the increasing popularity of collegiate nursing programs led the board of trustees to close the school officially in 1987. In 1988, the hospital established a clinical affiliation with the State University that continues today to provide clinical rotations for third- and fourth-year student nurses.

In 1970 the hospital, in cooperation with the Middleboro Trust Company, built Medical Office Park on land adjacent to the hospital's campus. This three-story medical office building was established as a condominium restricted to physicians with active medical staff privileges at MCH. To begin the enterprise the hospital leased sufficient land for the building and adjacent parking for 50 years to the condominium association and then constructed the medical office building on the leased land. Once all condominiums were sold, the hospital relinquished all title to the building, but it remains the leaseholder of the land. The Middleboro Trust Company holds mortgages for each condominium. Today, the building is totally owned and managed by the condominium association of physicians, a for-profit corporation. The hospital provides no services to Medical Office Park except for snow removal and general landscaping services at cost. Unless the hospital agrees to furnish additional land, Medical Office Park cannot be expanded. Currently all 30 offices are occupied. Each office has approximately 6,000 square feet. Its current assessed valuation for local tax purposes, done under a special provision in the local tax code, is $375,670 with a cap of 2 percent increase per tax year. Real estate appraisers have repeatedly stated that given its "limited and restricted use" they are unable to provide a fair market value. The current facility meets all current building codes. Over the years, individual condominiums have been sold to other members of MCH's active medical staff. The last sale in 2010 was estimated to be for $300,250.

Although tranquil in nature, this hospital has experienced volatile periods in its history. Since 1930, major disagreements between area physicians (MDs and DOs) created two independent systems in the community. Physicians trained in osteopathic medicine, for example, still continue to refer patients to other osteopathic physicians, often located in Capital City, even though local allopathic physicians (i.e., MDs) could manage the case.

Six years ago the board dismissed the president of MCH, who had served in this capacity for 31 years. The board of trustees cited no formal reasons, although it is known that the board refused to honor his request for a multiyear contract. The medical staff fully supported the termination of this individual. Five years ago James Higgens was appointed president.

The hospital has also experienced frequent staff changes in certain management positions. "Conflict with administration" is the most frequently cited reason for these resignations. Over the past 12 years no chief nursing officer has served for more than four years. Conflict with the medical staff involving patient care practices and administration concerning nurse scheduling and staffing levels, recently led to the resignation of Mary

Nurse, RN, after three years' service in this position. Nurse had worked for the hospital for 18 years at the time of her resignation. The vice president for nursing position is currently vacant. The director of education, Janet Martin, RN, is currently acting director of nursing. The administration accepted Nurse's resignation in stride and has told the board that she could not effectively manage the nursing department and communicate administration's policies to the nursing staff. Nurse did not support the decision to lower the staffing levels in nursing and the hiring of licensed practical nurses (LPNs) to replace registered nurses. While Nurse understood the need to reduce hospital expenses, she recommended that the hospital reorganize using small nursing units, each with a manager and support team. This plan was dismissed by the senior management team as too costly. The medical staff took no position on Nurse's resignation.

Nurse had been hired shortly before the nurses voted on unionization in 2010. In 2010, the petition to be recognized as a bargaining unit failed by the vote of 43 percent to 57 percent. Shortly before her resignation, however, Nurse had warned Higgens that another petition for another election was being discussed by nurses because of implications associated with downsizing the inpatient capacity of the hospital. Management's position for staff termination ignored seniority and emphasized "competency and job performance." On at least three occasions, terminated employees wrote to the local paper complaining that the hospital was looking to retain "only those workers who would work for less."

While members of the board were surprised by Nurse's resignation, all have expressed support for the current administration.

GOVERNANCE AND ORGANIZATION

The board of trustees is composed of 14 members, each elected for a four-year term. Elections are held at the annual meeting of the corporation. Nominees for trustees-at-large and trustee officers are chosen by the board nominating committee and presented to all hospital incorporators for consideration. Staggered terms of office ensure that no more than four new members are elected annually. The hospital's bylaws reserve two positions on the board for physicians nominated by the medical staff, but the rules specifically state that no physician nominated by the medical staff can be an elected officer of the board. Board members may succeed themselves. There are no limitations on the number of terms an individual can serve as a member of the board of trustees. Current board officers are as follows:

Rich has been board chairman for the past 12 years and has more than 16 years of service on the hospital board. His term will end next year. Steel has been vice chairman for 11 years and has more than 18 years of service on the board. His term will end this year. All other board members except Elton Giles have previously served at least one complete term as a trustee. Seed has recently informed the board that, given his business interests, he will be unable to serve another term.

The hospital's president (James Higgens) and the president of the medical staff (Frederick Mask, MD) are ex-officio members of the board of trustees. Standing committee of the board include the following:

Executive Committee	All board officers
Long-Range Planning	Steel (Chair), Paul, Land, and Simon
Finance	Meadows (Chair), Water, Corn, and Giles
Quality Assurance	Tracer (Chair), Seed, Wheat, and Mask
Nominating	Seed (Chair), Crop, and Rich

The board of trustees meets monthly. Prior to the annual meeting in March, a two-day retreat is held to review progress and update corporate plans. The executive committee meets with Higgens weekly and tours the hospital. Once every two years, each board member is sponsored by the hospital to participate in a continuing education program offered by either the American Hospital Association or the State Hospital Association.

A special ad hoc subcommittee of the board, staffed by John O'Hara, the hospital's chief financial officer, is examining its options for responding to physician requests for "more good inexpensive office space close to the hospital."

The board is currently considering a change in its bylaws to reduce the size of the board from 14 to 8 and increase the term of appointment to six years.

SENIOR MANAGEMENT TEAM

PRESIDENT

James Higgens holds an undergraduate degree in sociology and master's degree in hospital administration from a major midwestern university. Prior to becoming administrator, he completed a two-year postgraduate residency at Lake Shore Hospital (450 beds) in Chicago and was the chief operating officer at Capital City General Hospital in Capital City (365 beds) for many years. He served two years with the US Army Medical Service Corps in Europe.

A Fellow in the American College of Healthcare Executives (ACHE), Higgens is vice chairman of the board of directors of the State Hospital Association. He has authored several professional papers on hospital management and is noted for his ability to interact with the medical staff and his understanding of hospital operations.

When asked what he considers to be the major issues facing the hospital, he mentioned continued financial strength, long-range planning, cooperative ventures with the medical staff, increased worker productivity, and possible affiliation with another hospital or national chain of voluntary hospitals. He indicated that Webster Hospital, given its size, was no real threat to MCH. He also said that he has every confidence in the national search firm he has retained to fill the director of nursing position. When asked to describe the potential for union activities in the hospital, he stated, "Any movement in this direction should be curtailed when I find the right person to head up nursing."

When asked to describe MCH's primary strength, Higgens said there were two—the medical staff and the board. In contrast, when asked to list the primary threats, he indicated that less of the area's population appears to have adequate hospital insurance and that rates paid by the state for Medicaid and the federal government under Medicare were making it difficult to prosper. When asked his strategy to cope with these rates, he said, "It's simple. We will continue to strive for good inpatient occupancy and lower our operational costs throughout the hospital. Although the board has required that I bring all plans to them, they have generally approved everything." Although he was concerned that a national for-profit firm has recently purchased a hospital just east of Capital City, he sees no local consequences associated with this decision.

Quotes from his recent interview include "Our hospital wants to be the low-cost, high-quality provider in the area. We need to reduce our inpatient capacity in the future and be much more creative than we have been concerning physician recruitment and retention." When asked about the financial health of the hospital, Higgens said, "We are very conservative; we don't like to carry too much debt. While our building is getting old it is still modern, and we have the most up-to-date technology for patient and medical care."

Senior Vice President for Finance and Chief Financial Officer

John O'Hara has been employed in this position for nine years. His education includes an undergraduate degree in accounting from State University and a master's in business administration from an eastern university. He is a certified public accountant and an active member of the Healthcare Financial Management Association (HFMA). Previous positions include being vice president for finance for Seneca Hospital (NY) and assistant controller at two hospitals in New England. He has more than 25 years of professional experience.

Since arriving at the hospital, O'Hara has revised and updated many financial practices. On six different occasions he has received special commendations for excellence from the board, most recently for upgrading telecommunication services in the hospital at a reduced cost. When asked about future plans and priorities, he mentioned that the hospital needed a better financial information system that could link financial and patient care data; he is preparing a request for proposal for the management team to review and take to the board. He also mentioned that he believed that the hospital's relationship with Regional Blue Cross as well as other insurance companies would remain as harmonious as it has been in the past. O'Hara negotiates all contracts with physician professional associations (e.g., radiology) having a contractual relationship with the hospital. He has led hospital efforts to employ hospitalists beginning in 2012 and the selective purchase of medical practices by Medical Practices Subsidiary (MPS), Inc.

O'Hara recently reported that the most recent Centers for Medicare & Medicaid Services (CMS) calculated case mix index for the hospital was 1.5250. He indicated that MCH is following the pattern of most hospitals nationwide with this index increasing slightly over the past five years. He also mentioned the need for a budgetary process that was based on budgeted units of services in contrast to full-time equivalent (FTE) employees. O'Hara does not appear to be well liked by employees in the hospital. He has been responsible for the implementation of the hospital's plan to downsize its inpatient acute care capacity. Often he has been blamed by current and former employees for decisions to terminate or reassign staff in keeping with this plan, a plan he contributed to but that was designed and approved by Higgens and the board.

He is currently chairing a special management and medical staff committee to examine a hospital managed care plan (HMO or PPO) and different approaches to meet expectations established by recent federal legislation, including accountable care organizations. A report is expected in three months.

O'Hara serves as the chief financial officer for the hospital and reports to Higgens. He has responsibility for the hospital admitting department and the business office. He is also CEO of MPS, Inc., which owns and manages select medical practices of affiliated physicians. MPS is owned as a for-profit subsidiary of the hospital with its own board of directors.

O'Hara regularly attends all MCH board meetings.

SENIOR VICE PRESIDENT FOR INFORMATION SYSTEMS AND CHIEF INFORMATION OFFICER

Mabel Watkins was appointed to this position four years ago and is charged with implementing the new electronic medical records system. This system includes the hospital and all owned medical practices. Prior to joining the management team, Watkins was deputy CIO for a major medical center in a midwestern city. She was born in Jasper and earned her undergraduate degree in computer science at state university and MBA at a private eastern university. She has approximately 15 years' experience in hospital IT and is a member of the College of Healthcare Information Management Executives (CHIME). She manages all aspects of the internal information technology (IT) infrastructure and is also responsible for IT system security. She also co-chairs the hospital's task force on meaningful use.

When interviewed, Watkins stated, "Our electronic health record system is one of the reasons we have qualified for the maximum financial award every year since 2012 under the federal meaningful use criteria. Our system is changing how and what information we capture as well as our clinical and medical practice. Given the significant investment we made in acquiring and implementing the system it has to lower our operational costs. I believe it is beginning to show progress." Every year the hospital has participated in the federal meaningful use program, it has qualified for the maximum financial award. Watkins also indicated that some of her most difficult challenges include the number and types of vendor and service contracts her office manages, assessing the value of new technologies, and staying in compliance with regulations and best practices for securing protected health information (PHI). Direct reports include the department of medical records and the offices of IT systems services, IT grants and contracts, IT system security, and telecommunications.

VICE PRESIDENT FOR PROFESSIONAL SERVICES

Rob Stewart has held this position for 15 years. He had previously been assistant administrator for professional services for seven years. Stewart holds both an undergraduate and graduate degree in health administration from a southern university and is an active member of ACHE. He also served six years in the US Air Force Reserve (Medical Service Corps).

Stewart first came to MCH as part of his administrative residency requirement for his graduate degree. He has held a number of management positions in the hospital. During an interview, Stewart indicated that he had recently presented a plan to Higgens for the adoption of a formal guest relations program. He reports to Higgens and is responsible for the following departments:

- ◆ Dietary
- ◆ Pharmacy
- ◆ Physical therapy
- ◆ Occupational therapy
- ◆ Recreation therapy
- ◆ Speech therapy
- ◆ Social services
- ◆ All outpatient departments and services, including the emergency department.

He is also chairman of the hospital disaster planning committee and serves on committees of the State Hospital Association.

During a recent interview he expressed hope that the medical staff would become more realistic in their view of administration, and he felt that the hospital should seriously consider providing certain services off campus. While he indicated that he was disappointed that the hospital has elected not to provide contractual therapy services to area nursing homes—a plan he worked on for more than a year—he understood that "other priorities need attention first." He also indicated that "that past five years have been the most difficult" of his career and that too often "good employees had to be dismissed or reassigned because of the changes in the hospital sector." When asked to describe exactly what he does in the hospital, he said he spends most of his time working with department heads "in their offices," and he looks forward to his new project of establishing a more effective quality assurance/total quality management program.

Associate Vice President for Operations

Ted Beck joined MCH as a billing clerk when he graduated from high school 24 years ago. Since that time he has held positions as accounts receivable manager, director of purchasing, and most recently, director of the business office. He recently completed his undergraduate degree in health administration at State University. After the retirement of Hank Wrench last year, Beck was appointed assistant administrator for operations and promoted to associate administrator six months ago. Beck is a member of ACHE and plans to complete his certification exam within two years. For the past three years, employees have voted Beck the "Outstanding Supervisor." He is currently developing a plan for shared laundry services with area nursing homes.

He reports to Higgens and has responsibility for the following departments:

◆ Parking and security

◆ Engineering and maintenance

◆ Housekeeping

◆ Laundry

◆ Purchasing, materials management, and supply chain management

◆ Human resources

When interviewed, Beck indicated that he had just completed the plan and new job description for the director of human resources position, vacant since the recent resignation of Sally Simmons. Under his plan the new hire will be called the assistant administrator for human resources and will report directly to Higgens. Beck also indicated that, given the range of his current duties and associated details, he has just about enough time to check that each of his departments is running smoothly. Although he is busy, as acting director of human resources he does all exit interviews. When asked to characterize the nursing department, he expressed confidence that a new director in that department could solve any problems and that LPN substitution for RNs who resign has been an effective policy in curtailing financial increases.

Beck indicated that Simmons really resigned as director of human resources over the issue of outplacement services not being provided to terminated employees. Although Beck said that Simmons had a valid point regarding the hospital's responsibility to loyal employees, he supported O'Hara's position that MCH could not afford to spend money on employees it no longer needed. Beck also said human resources was a complex area that he did not fully understand, and he was looking forward to hiring a qualified replacement quickly.

It should also be noted that Beck has strongly urged MCH to affiliate with a national voluntary chain of hospitals to access joint purchasing services. His recent analysis shows that the hospital could save up to 8 percent on medical supplies if it were to change its purchasing affiliation to a large national chain. A consultant noted that the development of a state-of-the-art supply chain management program could lower inventory costs by 11 percent and reduce warehouse space by 25 percent. According to Beck, "Supply chain management needs to become a major priority."

Assistant Vice President for Human Resources

This newly created position is currently vacant. A regional search and consulting firm has been retained to identify qualified candidates. The hospital has indicated that it would consider changing this position to a vice president with direct report to Higgens. Sufficient funds have been budgeted to support this position and a small staff.

Vice President for Nursing

This position is currently vacant. A recruitment firm has been retained to identify qualified candidates. In addition to having a high degree of professional nursing experience, candidates must have demonstrated administrative talents. To date, no internal applications have been received. Two candidates identified by the recruitment firm were recently interviewed. One candidate withdrew before any decision could be made. The other was not retained based on her limited management experience. On recent consultation with the recruitment firm, Higgens informed the board that this position probably would remain vacant for at least another six months.

This position reports to the administrator and has responsibility for all in-patient nursing services in the hospital, including ICU/CCU and pediatrics, maternity, general medical–surgical services, and central surgical supply as well as the department of education.

Janet Martin, RN, director of education, is currently acting director of nursing. Martin has held her position as director of education for the past 20 years. She is a graduate of the Middleboro Community Hospital School of Nursing and holds an undergraduate degree in nursing and a master's degree in nursing education from State University. Combining 36 years' experience between nursing and education, Martin has held a variety of nursing positions at MCH, including staff nurse, charge nurse, evening nursing supervisor, and night nursing supervisor. On three different occasions, she has been acting director of nursing.

Martin knows every nurse in the hospital. She is very well liked and known to listen to her department heads, charge nurses, and head nurses. She indicated, however, that she still feels very uncomfortable with administration. While all department heads in nursing were relieved when Martin (again) agreed to become acting director, some indicated that Martin really was not qualified for the position on a permanent basis. One even stated, "She really doesn't have the ability to present our position. She just implements what administration tells her to do."

Martin recently informed Higgens that she would retire in six months.

The director of education is responsible for ensuring that all nurses remain proficient in professional practice. In-hospital seminars and workshops are provided. The director also serves as the liaison official with the nursing department and their student nurses from State University. In the past Martin has declined the opportunity to apply for the director of nursing position. When interviewed, she indicated that the hospital needs to listen to its nurses, attract a "good" director of nursing, and provide staff nurses more opportunity to influence patient care practices. Martin also said she "believes that team nursing, in contrast to primary nursing, was being forced on the hospital by the availability of qualified and experienced registered nurses and economics." She also indicated that she felt obligated to (again) become acting director of nursing to help the hospital.

The vice president for nursing reports to Higgens and supervises the following services:

- Pediatrics

- Maternity and nursery service

- All medical and surgical units

- ICU/CCU

- Nursing education and staff development

- Nursing quality assurance

◆ Case management services

◆ Central sterile supply

◆ Operating rooms

Until 2010, the vice president for nursing also managed all outpatient clinics and the emergency department. As part of the plan to downsize the inpatient capacity of the hospital and adjust to an increase in the demand for outpatient services, responsibility for these units was transferred to the associate administrator for professional services.

The vice president for nursing and the hospital's medical director, Dr. Fred Limpey, regularly convene the hospital's CMS Core Measures Working Group. Other members of the committee include Hazel Webster, RN, director of quality programs, and Candace Mathews, RN, director of case management. This group examines all CMS quality data furnished to the hospital by the area Quality Improvement Organization and institutes appropriate actions. This group also measures and monitors other specific quality measures. Eighteen months ago this group, working with a consultant, implemented a formal quality improvement program to prevent:

◆ Ventilator-associated pneumonia (VAP)

◆ Central line–associated bloodstream infection (CLABSI)

◆ Surgical wound infection (SWI)

Each program involved a specific bundle of services, policies, and procedures that constitute an evidence-based standard of care. For example, studies indicate that 5.3 CLABSIs occur in ICU per 1,000 catheter days and that approximately 18 percent of CLABSIs result in death. Studies indicate that VAP occurs in up to 15 percent of patients receiving mechanical ventilation. Whenever the bundle of required services, policies, and procedures is not fully implemented, the Core Measures Working Group determines the facts surrounding the case and reports its recommendations to the administrator for implementation. Frequently it must determine whether the problem is with a system or with a specific nurse or physician adhering to clinical protocols. Since implementing the standards, the occurrence of VAP, CLABSI, and SWI has declined by at least 65 percent.

SPECIAL ASSISTANT FOR PROFESSIONAL SERVICES

Marie Calley is a recent graduate of the health and hospital administration program (MBA) at a private eastern university. She has held this position for six months, having moved back to Middleboro nine months ago when her husband accepted a position with the law firm of Giles, Giles, and Drew. She reports directly to Higgens. Calley also holds an undergraduate degree in English. While in graduate school, she studied with one of the leading academic experts in hospital strategic planning. Her previous professional experience is limited to a two-year residency at Coastal Medical Center (450 beds) in a major western city. Calley recently applied for membership in ACHE.

Calley is responsible for the operation of three departments: radiology, laboratory, and anesthesiology. Based on a recent positive evaluation, Higgens has taken her off probation, a condition for any new employee. When interviewed, she indicated that she hopes to learn more about her departments and ensure that budgets are adhered to. Medical terminology and requests for new equipment she "really does not understand" have often sent her "back to the books," and she still seeks help from Higgens. She feels the hospital needs to develop a formal marketing program and says the physicians she deals with are clearly committed to the goals of the hospital.

Calley believes that other women employees perceive her as the "young professional woman role model" in the hospital, a status she says she is somewhat uncomfortable with. She feels she made the right decision to refer a group of concerned employees to Beck as acting director of human resources to share their views about the need for a day care program for dependents of hospital employees. She is a graduate of the local high school. When asked to characterize the hospital, she said it resembles a textbook case, "a 'good' hospital beginning to run itself as a 'good' business." While she understands the distress many employees feel about the recent changes in this hospital, she said that "most just do not understand, we have to adjust to changing demands and work cooperatively with our medical staff if we are to remain a viable hospital in the future."

DIRECTOR OF VOLUNTEER SERVICES/PUBLIC RELATIONS

Janet Stock has held this position for the last four years. She holds an undergraduate degree from State University and has previously served as director of volunteer efforts at the American Red Cross Chapter in Capital City. Stock is known for her ability to attract and retain volunteers from all facets of the community. Under her direction the hospital volunteer and auxiliary programs have been expanding.

She is also responsible for media relations and the preparation of the hospital's annual report. She reports to Higgens and has said if he reassigns her to report to anyone else, she will resign. When interviewed, she indicated that hospital volunteers were getting harder to find. She also noted that hospital advertising has limited her ability to place hospital stories in the local newspaper. The mayor of Middleboro recently awarded her a community citation for her demonstrated effort involving the Middleboro Hospital Baby Car Seat Program.

THE MEDICAL STAFF AND MEDICAL RESOURCES

The active medical staff has 172 physicians, and the general medical staff has 9 hospitalists. Physicians with "consulting" status on the medical staff must maintain "active" status at Capital City General Hospital, University Hospital in University Town, or another hospital. Appointment to the medical staff requires that the physician be board certified, unless granted a formal waiver based on 20 or more years of affiliation with MCH.

ANESTHESIOLOGY

The hospital maintains a contractual relationship with Anesthesiology Associates of Middleboro (PA) to provide all needed services. Dr. Frederick Mask is president of this professional association and chairperson of MCH's anesthesiology department.

EMERGENCY MEDICINE

The hospital maintains a contractual relationship with Emergency Medical Associates of Middleboro (PA) to provide all needed services. Dr. Simi Hines is president of this professional association and chairperson of this department.

DEPARTMENT OF FAMILY PRACTICE

This department includes physicians in private practice. Dr. Joe Apple is chairperson of this department.

DEPARTMENT OF INTERNAL MEDICINE

This department includes physicians in private practice in various specialties, including general internal medicine, pediatrics, allergy and immunology, cardiology, gastroenterology, ENT, psychiatry, oncology, and hematology. Dr. Godfrey Hurt is chairperson of this department.

DEPARTMENT OF PATHOLOGY

The hospital maintains a contractual relationship with Pathology Associates of Middleboro (PA) for all needed services. Dr. Douglas Mushroom is the president of this association and the chairperson of this department.

DEPARTMENT OF RADIOLOGY

The hospital maintains a contractual relationship with Radiology Associates of Middleboro (PA) for all needed services. Dr. Adam Picture is president of this association and the chairperson of this department.

DEPARTMENT OF SURGERY

This department includes physicians in private practice in various specialties. Dr. Limpey is the chairperson of this department.

DEPARTMENT OF HOSPITAL MEDICINE

The hospital currently employs nine physicians trained in internal medicine to provide in-house 24-hour care and services as hospitalists. Although hospitalists are members of the general medical staff and eligible for committee appointment, based on the medical staff bylaws hospitalists cannot admit nor vote on medical staff resolutions. Hospitalists are scheduled by the medical staff coordinator.

MEDICAL STAFF ORGANIZATION

Dr. Mask (department of anesthesiology) is president of the medical staff, a position he has held for the last two years. The president is elected every two years. No additional compensation is received for service as an elected officer of the medical staff. Dr. Carlos Leatros (department of pathology) is vice chair. At the last meeting of the medical staff, physicians currently located in the medical office building presented a letter asking that "the medical staff recommend to the hospital that the hospital work with the physician owners to upgrade and expand facilities and that the building be enlarged to accommodate even more members of the medical staff." After discussion it was decided that this issue was not a medical staff issue and that the current residents of the medical office building should directly communicate their request to Higgens.

Dr. Limpey (department of surgery) is employed part-time by the hospital as the medical director and chief medical officer. He provides staff support to all medical staff committees and assists the administrator on special projects. For example, he chairs the monthly meeting of the CMS Core Measures Working Group.

Standing committees of the medical staff include:

◆ Bylaws Committee

◆ Cancer Committee

- Credentials Committee

- Critical Care Committee

- Education Committee

- Emergency Services Committee

- Executive Committee

- Hospitalist Practice Committee

- Medical Records Committee

- Pharmacy and Therapeutics Committee

- Quality Assurance Committee

- Tissue/Transfusion Committee

- Utilization Review Committee

The executive committee of the medical staff meets monthly or as needed. Other committees meet monthly. The entire medical staff meets quarterly. Recredentialing is done at the annual meeting of the medical staff.

Dr. Raymond Samuels (pediatrics) has recently written to the medical staff indicating that he would like to be considered for election as president. Without criticizing the performance of the incumbent, Samuels wrote that the interests of the medical staff would be better represented by a physician in private practice, not a physician in a hospital-based practice such as anesthesiology.

OTHER INFORMATION

EMERGENCY DEPARTMENT SPECIAL STUDY

The hospital has just received a report from the Department of Health Services Management at State University that included the following information on the MCH emergency department.

Emergency Department Demand by Day of Week	Percent
Sunday	22.3
Monday	13.2
Tuesday	9.2
Wednesday	7.2
Thursday	9.0
Friday	12.8
Saturday	26.3

Demand by Time of Day	
12:00–2:00 a.m.	12.5
2:00–4:00 a.m.	9.8
4:00–6:00 a.m.	5.9
6:00–8:00 a.m.	9.6
8:00–10:00 a.m.	3.7
10:00 a.m.–12:00 p.m.	2.3
12:00–2:00 p.m.	3.5
2:00–4:00 p.m.	4.2
4:00–6:00 p.m.	7.6
6:00–8:00 p.m.	9.5
8:00–10:00 p.m.	12.6
10:00 p.m.–12:00 a.m.	18.8

Source: Three-month study, 12/31/CY

Type of ED Care %	3:00 p.m.–11:00 p.m.	11:00 p.m.–7:00 a.m.	7:00 a.m.–3:00 p.m.
Emergency	3.1	12.5	4.4
Urgent	32.6	36.2	48.3
Nonurgent	64.3	51.3	47.3
Total	100	100	100

Emergency Department Patients by Age (%)	Male	Female
Under 15	14.4	10.4
15–24	11.4	7.8
25–44	19.6	14.0
45–64	6.4	6.4
65–74	1.7	2.3
75 and older	1.5	4.1
Total	55	45

Source: Three-month study, 12/31/CY

This study also documented the growing problem associated with psychotic patients and other patients in need of acute mental health services. Frequently these patients must wait in the emergency department for extended periods of time before they can be transferred to appropriate service providers. The state hospital in Capital City is the closest facility that accepts involuntary emergency admissions. Local services only provide outpatient services. The report documents that within the past year, four patients waited more than three days in the emergency department before transfer and on five days, mental health patients awaiting transfer occupied 12 of the emergency department's 27 beds.

This information was collected as part of a pilot study to determine appropriate emergency services in communities served by two or more emergency departments. This study suggests that current operational costs in the emergency department are approximately 18 percent above costs incurred in similar hospitals with similar utilization. During 2014, approximately 12 percent of emergency department visits resulted in a hospital admission.

RESULTS OF THE BOARD RETREAT

Approximately six weeks ago, the board and senior management team gathered for a special two-day strategic review of the hospital. Strategic Visions, Inc., facilitated the retreat sessions. The retreat was organized after board chair Michael Rich and vice chair Peter Steel each attended a national meeting of the American Hospital Association on strategic options for community hospitals. Both Rich and Steel returned from this meeting with specific questions regarding whether the hospital should develop off-campus services, acquire and operate additional medical practices, and affiliate with other service providers, including the possibility of an asset merger or sale to a for-profit corporation. Given the nature of topics discussed, the board has agreed not to publicly discuss these topics until the full board has had the opportunity "to better understand and address the strategic options it faces." The board has asked that management continue to assess the implications of the Sarbanes-Oxley Act and other relevant laws and regulations on hospital governance.

The board, meeting without senior managers, also discussed whether the compensation package for the president should include financial incentives linked to financial and quality measures. The board agreed to continue this discussion and has asked the state hospital association for examples of contracts used at other similar hospitals. The retreat served to convey to the entire board the significance of these issues as well as other issues it faced, including the following:

CHANGE IN CERTIFICATE OF NEED LAW

Harry Water, a trustee and an elected member of the state legislature, has been asked by the governor to introduce legislation that would deregulate the healthcare system and allow the current Certificate of Need (CON) law to lapse at the end of 2016. Water has shared with the board that he feels that, with the governor's endorsement, this legislation would be successful. He is concerned, however, that the demise of this legislation would allow hospitals and other currently regulated healthcare providers to move into new markets, such as Jasper. Water also shared with the board that he feels the governor could be convinced to delay the demise of the CON law until the end of at least 2018 if he were furnished with compelling reasons.

The leadership of the hospitals in Capital City and other major cities in the state strongly support the demise of the current CON laws and the community hospitals in suburban and rural areas generally want the law retained.

Water has asked the board for its views on this law and has asked Higgens to furnish the entire board with a legal opinion on whether federal antitrust laws and regulations would constrain other hospitals from attempting to serve Jasper and other communities traditionally served by MCH. Higgens has asked the hospital counsel—Giles, Giles, and Drew—to furnish this opinion within 60 days. The state hospital association has reserved any judgment on the CON law until "after the specific legislation has been introduced." Higgens reported that he felt that this association will be unable to present a unified position given the split sentiments of its constituents on this statute.

SINGLE-OCCUPANCY INPATIENT ROOMS

Higgens has suggested the hospital hire a consulting firm to assess whether single-occupancy inpatient rooms are possible and desirable. He feels that it would give the hospital an advantage over its competition without any significant changes in staffing or expenses if the hospital implemented such a plan over a five- to seven-year period. When he presented this idea to the board he indicated that inpatient hospital admissions rates were continuing to drop and average length of stay also was stable or dropping, indicating that a larger number of hospital rooms could be configured for single occupancy. The board wants to consider this idea. Note that current double-occupancy rooms dedicated to maternity services can be modernized for $100,000 each, regardless of whether they are to be single or double occupancy. Current medical surgical rooms can be converted to single- or double-occupancy birthing rooms for $115,000.

STRATEGIC VISIONS' RECOMMENDATION

Strategic Visions, Inc., recommended that the hospital consider developing a 25-bed critical access hospital and rural health center in Harris City to serve Harris City, Minortown, and Carterville. Such a facility could meet the federal requirements of the Medicare Rural Hospital Flexibility Program. The 25 beds would be dual-licensed as acute swing beds. The adjacent rural health clinic could house primary care physicians directly employed by the hospital. Higgens has not yet taken this suggestion to the board.

MEDICAL OFFICE BUILDING OPTIONS

The attorney managing the estate of the landowner (who originally leased the land to the hospital) has recently informed the hospital that this land will be bequeathed to the hospital as a result of the owner's death last month. This move creates a series of options, as the land and structures could be exempt from local taxes once they are owned by the hospital. O'Hara is currently developing a series of options to be considered.

IRS 990 DISCLOSURES

The recent release of the IRS Form 990 indicates that the 2014 salaries for the ten highest paid hospital employees are as follows:

James Higgens	President	$659,600
John O'Hara	Senior vice president for finance/CFO	313,000
Mabel Watkins	Senior vice president for information systems/CIO	303,450
Janet Martin	Director, nursing—acting	181,500
Dr. Martin Shine	Hospitalist	212,445
Dr. William Lewis	Hospitalist	198,445
Dr. Mega Gupta	Hospitalist	178,320
Dr. Cathy Frost	Hospitalist	177,540
Dr. Fred Limpey	Chief medical officer	155,000
Martha Limpey	Director, medical records	113,140

Compensation also includes benefits that average 34 percent above salary. Note that emergency services, radiology, pathology, and anesthesiology are provided by contract. Currently the hospital does not directly employ any physicians in these specialties.

The hospital has ownership interests in 25 physician practices. MCH Medical Practices Subsidiary, Inc., a wholly owned for-profit subsidiary of the hospital, employs all physicians and staff used in these practices.

Additional information regarding MCH's staffing, utilization, payer mix, financial status, and patient demographics may be found in the following tables.

TABLE 5.1

Medical Staff
Information as of
December 2014

Name	Notes	Office	Age	Specialty	2014 Patient Days
Family Practice: Active Staff					
F. Player		5	70	General Practice	235
G. Banero		8	55	General Practice	319
J. Apple		6	59	General Practice	174
S. Fistru		7	58	General Practice	260
S. Mix		2	64	General Practice	130
Family Practice: Consulting Staff					
C. Berrnally		3	38	General Practice*	101
D. Mathews		3	45	General Practice*	48
H. Cavenero		3	55	General Practice*	57
H. Wang		3	40	General Practice	79
J. Yates		3	44	General Practice	51
N. Chamerberlin		3	47	General Practice	118
S. Mathews		3	42	General Practice	18
Internal Medicine					
A. Barton	MA	1	45	Internal Medicine	812
B. Crush		3	63	Internal Medicine	380
C. Douglas	MA	1	41	Internal Medicine	800
D. Justin		1	67	Internal Medicine	310
D. Meow		1	60	Internal Medicine	280
D. Michael		4	45	Internal Medicine*	250
E. Frost	MA	3	41	Internal Medicine	490
F. Grist		3	50	Internal Medicine	140
G. Filly		1	58	Internal Medicine	240
G. Hurt		8	55	Internal Medicine*	172

(continued)

Name	Notes	Office	Age	Specialty	2014 Patient Days
H. Hippster		1	56	Internal Medicine	250
J. Justin		4	59	Internal Medicine*	84
J. Vogel		5	55	Internal Medicine	103
K. Kessler	MA	1	34	Internal Medicine	658
L. Lesko	MA	1	38	Internal Medicine	560
L. Nask		5	56	Internal Medicine	203
M. Horse		1	68	Internal Medicine*	544
M. Mast		2	41	Internal Medicine	877
M. Master	MA	1	40	Internal Medicine	472
N. Nostrom		2	57	Internal Medicine	112
O. Ogg		2	39	Internal Medicine	572
P. Xiao		2	50	Internal Medicine	126
P. Trip		6	52	Internal Medicine	263
Q. Quinn		6	63	Internal Medicine	156
S. Jessey		7	60	Internal Medicine	177
S. Knach		8	67	Internal Medicine*	63
S. Steel		3	50	Internal Medicine	416
S. Stocapy		3	57	Internal Medicine	150
T. Beata		3	60	Internal Medicine	80
T. Cushing		3	62	Internal Medicine	87
T. Davis		3	58	Internal Medicine	203
T. Figher		3	54	Internal Medicine	306
T. King		3	63	Internal Medicine	64
Pediatrics					
A. Sloan		1	54	Pediatrics*	56
B. Bickford		1	50	Pediatrics	92
G. Gavin		1	44	Pediatrics	44

(continued)

Name	Notes	Office	Age	Specialty	2014 Patient Days
M. Miller	MA	3	40	Pediatrics	103
M. Bill		3	59	Pediatrics	52
N. Otter	MA	3	37	Pediatrics	105
O. Pushy		1	50	Pediatrics	120
P. Kettel		3	57	Pediatrics	70
P. Quester	MA	3	40	Pediatrics	280
Q. Reaper	MA	1	59	Pediatrics	81
R. Samuels	MA	1	47	Pediatrics	114
S. St. James	MA	1	40	Pediatrics	120
T. Turtle		1	58	Pediatrics*	240
U. Unvey	MA	3	56	Pediatrics	234
V. Vesh		1	52	Pediatrics*	92
W. Warren		1	56	Pediatrics*	84
W. Washed		3	64	Pediatrics	48
Allergy and Immunology					
S. Sleek		1	49	Allergy/Immunology	448
T. Gustave		1	53	Allergy/Immunology	207
T. Hampshire		3	58	Allergy/Immunology	204
Cardiology					
D. Eastman		1	56	Cardiology*	384
G. Hurst		1	60	Cardiology*	234
J. Dufresne		3	60	Cardiology	180
T. Underwood	MA	1	46	Cardiology	652
U. Victem		1	41	Cardiology*	471

TABLE 5.1
Medical Staff
Information as of
December 2014
(continued)

(continued)

Name	Notes	Office	Age	Specialty	2014 Patient Days
Gastroenterology					
T. Amas		1	60	Gastroenterology	120
T. Eisher		1	55	Gastroenterology	128
T. Tiger		2	59	Gastroenterology	58
T. Wingate		2	64	Gastroenterology	86
Y. Zaller		1	49	Gastroenterology	1,270
Z. Autumn	MA	1	44	Gastroenterology	748
Psychiatry					
A. Actor		1	42	Psychiatry	480
B. Banana		1	50	Psychiatry	432
F. Jilley		1	39	Psychiatry	360
I. Stanzl		2	61	Psychiatry	86
S. Zeus		2	40	Psychiatry	272
Other: Medicine					
C. Tunsteb		1	60	ENT	80
M. White		1	63	ENT	68
M. Whittier		1	44	ENT	353
V. Weckenson	MA	1	44	ENT	470
W. Xerox	MA	1	42	ENT	497
X. Yalper		1	57	ENT	170
B. Divan		1	44	Oncology/Hemo	440
M. Schoen		1	39	Oncology/Hemo*	401
S. Hatcher		1	53	Oncology/Hemo*	459
T. Kwok		1	32	Oncology/Hemo	150
C. Carp		3	54	ENT	300
F. Fish		3	49	ENT	280

(continued)

Name	Notes	Office	Age	Specialty	2014 Patient Days
Surgery: Orthopedic					
D. Jones		1	57	Orthopedic	1,376
G. Hooper		1	50	Orthopedic	1,253
K. Amberson		1	55	Orthopedic	1,540
K. Matthews		1	45	Orthopedic	1,721
K. Questrom	MA	1	39	Orthopedic	1,401
L. Rex		1	57	Orthopedic	1,703
M. Dillon		1	64	Orthopedic	1,420
M. Stanley	MA	1	49	Orthopedic	1,507
Surgery: General					
B. Hersh	MA	1	40	General	1,200
C. Isherum		1	57	General*	1,245
D. Jackson	MA	1	39	General	734
F. Limpey		1	58	General*	1,300
G. Munson		1	50	General*	586
H. Never	MA	1	45	General	870
I. O'Connell	MA	1	49	General	416
J. Putter	MA	1	62	General	601
J. Timas		1	59	General*	1,246
J. Victor		1	57	General*	980
Surgery: OB/GYN					
D. Dustin	MA	1	33	OB/GYN	650
E. Eberle		1	51	OB/GYN	290
F. Fraser		1	65	OB/GYN*	480
G. Gost	MA	1	45	OB/GYN	720
J. Kim		1	57	OB/GYN	336

TABLE 5.1
Medical Staff
Information as of
December 2014
(continued)

(continued)

Name	Notes	Office	Age	Specialty	2014 Patient Days
I. Japen		1	56	OB/GYN*	236
K. Lights		1	55	OB/GYN	186
M. Nester		1	59	OB/GYN*	280
Surgery: Other					
B. Bernal		1	45	Neuro	329
C. Eason	MA	1	56	Urology	450
D. Crow		1	50	Neuro	334
D. Fixer	MA	1	43	Urology	578
F. Seimer		1	59	Neuro	444
G. Tho		1	42	Plastic	332
H. Yee		1	58	Plastic	101
J. Underside		1	55	Thoracic	921
J. Warren		1	60	Thoracic	844
J. Yellow		1	60	General	640
J. Zetias		1	66	General	225
L. Clock		1	47	Thoracic	340
L. David		1	51	Vascular	310
L. Fession		1	44	Bariatric	380
L. Frederick		1	47	Vascular	340
M. Blue		1	46	Eye	300
M. Mold		1	45	Urology	650
N. Nerve		1	51	Urology	850
Department of Medicine: Consulting Staff					
W. Pokorny		9	51	Psychiatry	14
B. Rubble		3	54	Oncology	32
F. Feada		9	63	Hematology	32

(continued)

Name	Notes	Office	Age	Specialty	2014 Patient Days
F. Flint		9	56	Oncology	54
H. Ruth		9	42	Gastroenterology	65
J. Klock	MA	3	49	OB/GYN	130
K. Kipstein	MA	3	50	Cardiology	201
L. Gomez		9	44	Allergy	26
L. Mustard	MA	3	39	OB/GYN	223
M. McVoy		9	37	Psychiatry	32
O. Maeer	MA	3	42	Cardiology	133
P. Carles		9	60	Pulmonary Medicine	28
S. Ange		9	48	Endocrinology	84
S. Lott		9	50	Hematology	112
S. Malone		9	55	Allergy	31
S. Parish		9	48	Dermatology	16
V. Vitter		9	57	Hematology	102
Department of Surgery: Consulting Staff					
A. Hamp		9	48	General	45
A. Steve	MA	3	47	Thoracic	80
C. Finn	MA	3	49	Thoracic	39
F. Mike		9	60	Orthopedic	28
J. Wingate		9	50	Pediatric	30
L. Picture	MA	3	47	Orthopedic	76
L. Richard		9	45	Orthopedic	19
N. New		9	58	Orthopedic	24
S. Lee	MA	3	40	Orthopedic	56

TABLE 5.1
Medical Staff
Information as of
December 2014
(continued)

(continued)

Name	Notes	Office	Age	Specialty	2014 Patient Days
Department of Pathology: Active Staff					
A. Mixture		1	61	Pathology	
B. Nerverto		1	56	Pathology	
C. Leatros		1	47	Pathology	
D. Mushroom		1	42	Pathology	
D. Pathos		1	56	Pathology	
E. Fisher		1	54	Pathology	
F. Mautz		1	64	Pathology	
G. Wingate		1	63	Pathology	
Department of Radiology: Active Staff					
A. Picture		1	56	Radiology	
B. Quadic		1	45	Radiology	
C. Roetgen		1	61	Radiology	
D. Sunshine		1	40	Radiology	
M. Ray		1	45	Radiology	
K. Hines		1	50	Radiology	
W. Hines		1	39	Radiology	
L. Jinks		1	45	Radiology	
P. Patel		1	52	Radiology	
R. Ricker		1	34	Radiology	
R. El-Amin		1	44	Radiology	
R. Trippe		1	49	Radiology	
E. Tracer		1	49	Radiology	
Department of Anesthesiology: Active Staff					
A. Aaron		1	38	Anesthesiology	
B. Carter		1	62	Anesthesiology	

(continued)

Name	Notes	Office	Age	Specialty	2014 Patient Days
B. Dexter		1	66	Anesthesiology	
B. Harrington		1	63	Anesthesiology	
B. Nelson		1	60	Anesthesiology	
B. Thomas		1	64	Anesthesiology	
C. Fisher		1	54	Anesthesiology	
D. Gass		1	48	Anesthesiology	
E. Lister		1	61	Anesthesiology	
F. Mask		1	59	Anesthesiology	
Department of Emergency Medicine: Active Staff					
R. Romanikova		1	29	Emergency	
S. Hines		1	60	Emergency	
B. Casey		1	44	Emergency	
J. Smooth		1	54	Emergency	
G. Goodspeed		1	70	Emergency	
L. Jinks		1	45	Emergency	
M. Gotlike		1	52	Emergency	
J. Ishabi		1	43	Emergency	
L. Cytesmith		1	60	Emergency	
M. Welby		1	56	Emergency	
R. Hotlick		1	58	Emergency	
S. Tobias		1	51	Emergency	
Department of Hospital Medicine					
A. Palmer		1	32	Hospitalist	
B. Carlos		1	40	Hospitalist	
C. Frost		1	39	Hospitalist	
F. Drudge		1	35	Hospitalist	

TABLE 5.1
Medical Staff Information as of December 2014 (continued)

(continued)

TABLE 5.1
Medical Staff
Information as of
December 2014
(continued)

Name	Notes	Office	Age	Specialty	2014 Patient Days
M. Gupta		1	40	Hospitalist	
M. Shine		1	43	Hospitalist	
S. Ruderbacker		1	56	Hospitalist	
V. Martinez		1	44	Hospitalist	
W. Lewis		1	50	Hospitalist	

NOTES:

MA = Medical Associates

Office Location: 1=Middleboro; 2=Mifflenville; 3=Jasper; 4=Harris City; 5=Statesville; 6=Carterville; 7=Boalsburg; 8=Minortown; 9=Capital City; 10=Other

* = Medical practice owned by Medical Practice Subsidary (MPS), Inc.

(This table can also be found online at ache.org/books/Middleboro.)

TABLE 5.2
Hospital Inpatient
Occupancy by
Service,
2008–2014

Hospital Service	2014	2013	2012	2011	2010	2009	2008
Pediatrics							
Beds	12	14	16	18	18	18	18
Patient days	2,249	2,245	2,224	2,270	2,546	3,260	3,150
Occupancy	51.3%	43.9%	38.1%	34.6%	38.8%	49.6%	47.9%
Maternity							
Beds	26	28	28	29	29	29	29
Patient days	4,372	4,423	4,134	5,045	6,023	6,007	6,045
Occupancy	46.1%	43.3%	40.5%	47.7%	56.9%	56.8%	57.1%
Medical Surgical I							
Beds	50	50	50	50	50	50	50
Patient days	13,756	13,505	13,333	13,340	12,103	12,400	12,547
Occupancy	75.4%	74.0%	73.1%	73.1%	66.3%	67.9%	68.8%

(continued)

TABLE 5.2
Hospital Inpatient Occupancy by Service, 2008–2014 (continued)

Hospital Service	2014	2013	2012	2011	2010	2009	2008
Medical Surgical II							
Beds	50	50	50	50	50	50	50
Patient days	13,845	13,604	13,503	12,056	12,440	10,378	10,501
Occupancy	75.9%	74.5%	74.0%	66.1%	68.2%	56.9%	57.5%
Medical Surgical III							
Beds	44	50	53	55	55	53	53
Patient days	10,054	10,450	11,004	11,856	11,420	11,890	11,945
Occupancy	62.6%	57.3%	56.9%	59.1%	56.9%	61.5%	61.7%
Medical Surgical IV							
Beds	40	40	45	50	50	50	50
Patient days	9,850	9,893	9,833	10,956	11,584	12,282	12,470
Occupancy	67.5%	67.8%	59.9%	60.0%	63.5%	67.3%	68.3%
ICU/CCU							
Beds	18	18	18	18	18	20	20
Patient days	4,644	4,847	4,856	4,934	4,926	5,102	5,008
Occupancy	70.7%	73.8%	73.9%	75.1%	75.0%	69.9%	68.6%
Total Hospital							
Beds	240	250	260	270	270	270	270
Patient days	58,770	58,967	58,887	60,457	61,042	61,319	61,666
Occupancy	67.1%	65.5%	62.9%	62.2%	62.8%	63.1%	63.4%

(This table can also be found online at ache.org/books/Middleboro.)

TABLE 5.3

Detailed Utilization Statistics for 2014 and 2013

2014	Discharges	Patient Days	Inpatient Surgery	Outpatient Surgery	Births	ED Visits	ED Admits	OPV
January	890	4,959	201	362	98	2,134	272	9,558
February	823	4,655	209	350	84	1,883	238	8,973
March	934	5,098	190	372	101	2,090	268	9,495
April	956	5,124	193	348	112	2,063	254	9,088
May	923	5,170	197	394	109	2,110	283	9,265
June	1,025	5,768	185	345	108	2,203	260	8,857
July	897	4,535	170	325	99	2,083	253	9,436
August	862	4,425	165	303	101	2,068	250	9,356
September	898	4,978	187	365	109	2,205	275	9,030
October	893	4,990	198	323	114	2,003	245	9,234
November	863	4,923	193	395	104	2,209	249	9,345
December	766	4,145	170	302	109	2,027	240	8,245
Total	**10,730**	**58,770**	**2,258**	**4,184**	**1,248**	**25,078**	**3,087**	**109,882**
2013								
January	882	4,703	191	390	109	2,167	270	8,951
February	837	4,780	190	331	110	2,107	265	8,094
March	893	5,149	207	387	113	2,278	289	9,092
April	967	5,547	215	367	109	2,678	365	9,234
May	980	5,320	199	346	110	2,398	310	9,245
June	1,005	5,756	204	361	111	2,351	270	9,345
July	823	3,701	187	302	103	2,278	280	9,832
August	812	4,301	160	296	102	2,056	263	9,257
September	934	5,734	188	379	116	2,556	289	9,934
October	954	5,134	193	384	111	2,044	240	10,109
November	848	4,775	196	382	103	2,196	279	9,887
December	703	4,067	178	312	113	2,286	288	8,750
Total	**10,638**	**58,967**	**2,308**	**4,237**	**1,310**	**27,395**	**3,408**	**111,730**

NOTES:
ED Visits = Total emergency department visits
ED Admits = ED visits that lead to an inpatient admission
OPV = Outpatient Visits, excludes ED visits

(This table can also be found online at ache.org/books/Middleboro.)

	2014	2013	2012
Revenue			
Patient services revenue, total	**658,351,925**	**650,578,354**	**650,829,412**
Inpatient	312,565,340	315,343,506	322,465,856
Outpatient	345,786,585	335,234,848	328,363,556
Allowances and uncollectables—inpatient	200,564,989	190,282,353	185,374,561
Allowances and uncollectables—outpatient	203,464,546	200,343,595	196,294,375
Total	404,029,535	390,625,948	381,668,936
Net service revenue	**254,322,390**	**259,952,406**	**269,160,476**
Other operating revenue	154,229	288,354	372,343
Total operating revenue	**254,476,619**	**260,240,760**	**269,532,819**
Expenses			
Operating expenses			
Patient care services	80,373,449	78,354,002	77,343,526
Other professional services	69,363,454	68,394,262	68,001,200
General services	40,383,464	42,393,446	44,627,308
Fiscal and admin services	40,228,343	45,383,557	50,526,303
Interest	3,956,433	3,825,354	3,800,240
Depreciation	14,378,565	15,340,272	16,340,229
Community education and outreach	542,383	599,454	535,495

TABLE 5.4
Statement of Revenue and Expenses for Calendar Years Ending December 31 ($)

(continued)

TABLE 5.4

Statement of Revenue and Expenses for Calendar Years Ending December 31 ($) (continued)

	2014	2013	2012
Total operating expenses	249,226,091	254,290,347	261,174,301
Net income from operations	5,250,528	5,950,413	8,358,518
Nonoperating revenue			
Unrestricted gifts and bequests	76,342	147,841	111,343
Income from investments	1,978,564	2,018,334	3,005,264
Miscellaneous nonpatient revenue	118,453	134,575	157,394
Total	2,173,359	2,166,175	3,116,607
Nonoperating expenses	1,553,675	1,494,303	1,324,556
Net nonoperating income	619,684	671,872	1,792,051
Profit (loss)	5,870,212	6,622,285	11,475,125

(This table can also be found online at ache.org/books/Middleboro.)

TABLE 5.5

Balance Sheet as of December 31, 2012–2014 ($)

	2014	2013	2012
Current assets			
Cash	16,008,364	16,343,949	10,438,282
Short term investments	6,546,791	3,283,445	3,029,393
Accounts receivable—gross	72,564,867	71,540,304	70,283,443
Allowances for uncollectables	28,453,998	29,474,665	29,117,273
Accounts receivable—net	44,110,869	42,065,639	41,166,170
Due from third-party payers	378,559	349,228	103,450
Inventories	2,663,265	2,995,394	2,235,119
Prepaid expenses	89,020	72,343	69,372
Total current assets	69,796,868	65,109,998	57,041,786

(continued)

	2014	2013	2012
Noncurrent assets			
Property, plant, and equipment—gross	354,783,292	354,282,404	360,283,443
Less accumulated depreciation	176,453,887	171,133,779	165,242,577
Property, plant, and equipment—net	178,329,405	183,148,625	195,040,866
Other investments	39,997,354	39,105,569	34,674,187
Total assets	**288,123,627**	**287,364,192**	**286,756,839**
Current liabilities			
Accounts payable	16,342,575	15,369,594	16,002,347
Accrued salaries and wages	10,453,274	8,259,669	7,345,002
Accrued interest	134,569	156,304	700,585
Other accrued expenses	1,393,253	1,657,330	1,435,020
Due to third-party vendors	1,205,494	1,723,657	582,491
Long-term debt due within one year	5,142,939	4,920,338	4,823,293
Total current liabilities	**34,672,104**	**32,086,892**	**30,888,738**
Long-term debt	67,540,223	75,330,404	82,374,337
Total liabilities	**102,212,327**	**107,417,296**	**113,263,075**
Net assets			
Restricted	6,128,484	6,034,292	6,203,445
Unrestricted	179,782,816	179,782,816	179,782,816
Total net assets	**185,911,300**	**185,817,108**	**185,986,261**
Net assets + liabilities	288,123,627	293,234,404	299,249,336

TABLE 5.5
Balance Sheet as of December 31, 2012–2014 ($) (continued)

(This table can also be found online at ache.org/books/Middleboro.)

DRG Name	Number of Discharges					
	2014	**2013**	**2012**	**2011**	**2010**	**2009**
Normal newborn[1]	1,284	1,236	1,182	1,204	992	1,075
Vaginal delivery, no complications	943	898	858	874	720	781
Atherosclerosis	770	726	674	576	401	576
Caesarean section	356	351	336	342	282	306
Major joint or reattachment of lower extremity	301	314	327	364	287	364
Simple pneumonia and pleurisy	300	286	319	354	278	353
Chest pain	292	290	296	328	275	339
Chronic obstructive pulmonary disease	205	167	285	265	238	329
Acute myocardial infarction	195	165	197	197	236	275
Spinal fusion	139	157	165	175	230	241
Total top ten, excluding births	**3,501**	**3,354**	**3,457**	**3,475**	**2,947**	**3,564**
Total discharges	**10,730**	**10,638**	**10,243**	**10,733**	**10,040**	**10,238**
Percent top ten, excluding births	**32.63%**	**31.53%**	**33.75%**	**32.38%**	**29.35%**	**34.81%**

NOTE: 1. Counted as births, not discharges

TABLE 5.7
Patient Days by Type and Type of Payer, Percent of Total, 2014

Type of Patient Day	Total Patient Days	Medicare	Medicaid	BC HMO	BC PPO	BC Indemnity	Swift	CS PPO	Comm HMO	Comm PPO	Comm Indemnity	Other	Self Pay
Medical	43.1%	16.2%	2.8%	1.0%	0.2%	4.3%	0.8%	0.7%	2.1%	3.0%	10.0%	0.2%	1.8%
Surgical													
Nonorthopedic	22.1%	10.8%	2.8%	0.0%	1.0%	3.5%	0.2%	0.3%	0.9%	0.0%	1.6%	0.2%	0.8%
Orthopedic	10.7%	3.8%	2.7%	0.1%	0.3%	1.0%	0.2%	0.2%	0.6%	0.0%	1.6%	0.0%	0.2%
OB	7.5%	0.0%	2.0%	0.2%	0.2%	1.3%	0.1%	0.1%	0.6%	0.2%	1.7%	0.2%	0.9%
Newborn	4.3%	0.0%	1.1%	0.0%	0.2%	0.9%	0.0%	0.0%	0.3%	0.1%	1.0%	0.1%	0.6%
Other pediatric	3.8%	0.0%	0.6%	0.2%	0.1%	1.1%	0.1%	0.1%	0.1%	0.2%	1.1%	0.0%	0.2%
ICU/CCU	7.9%	6.0%	0.2%	0.0%	0.3%	0.2%	0.0%	0.1%	0.0%	0.0%	0.7%	0.2%	0.2%
Psychological	0.2%	0.1%	0.0%	0.0%	0.0%	0.0%	0.0%	0.1%	0.0%		0.0%	0.0%	0.0%
Substance abuse													
Detox	0.1%	0.0%	0.0%	0.0%	0.0%	0.0%	0.0%	0.0%	0.0%	0.0%	0.0%	0.0%	0.1%
Rehab	0.3%	0.0%	0.0%	0.0%	0.0%	0.0%	0.0%	0.0%	0.0%	0.0%	0.0%	0.0%	0.3%
Total	100.0%	36.9%	12.2%	1.5%	2.3%	12.3%	1.4%	1.6%	4.6%	3.5%	17.7%	0.9%	5.1%

NOTE: BC = Blue Cross
CS = Central States Good Health Network
Swift = Swift Health Plan
Comm = Commercial

Category	CMS Core Measure	State Benchmark	MCH 2014	MCH 2013	MCH 2012
Timely Heart Attack Care	Average number of minutes before outpatient with chest pain or possible heart attack who needed specialized care was transferred to another hospital	1 hr	n/a	n/a	n/a
Timely Heart Attack Care	Average number of minutes before outpatients with chest pain or possible heart attack got an ECG	8 min	9 min	n/a	n/a
Timely Heart Attack Care	Outpatients with chest pain or possible heart attack who got aspirin within 24 hours of arrival	100%	92%	90%	81%
Timely Heart Attack Care	Heart attack patients given PCI within 90 minutes of arrival	94%	96%	94%	94%
Effective Heart Attack Care	Heart attack patients given aspirin at discharge	100%	100%	100%	100%
Effective Heart Attack Care	Heart attack patients given a prescription for a statin at discharge	97%	98%	98%	94%
Effective Heart Failure Care	Heart failure patients given discharge instructions	92%	98%	94%	94%
Effective Heart Failure Care	Heart failure patients given an evaluation of left ventricular systolic (LVS) function	97%	94%	94%	95%
Effective Heart Failure Care	Heart failure patients given ACE inhibitor or ARB for left ventricular systolic dysfunction (LVSD)	97%	96%	95%	85%

(continued)

Category	CMS Core Measure	State Benchmark	MCH 2014	MCH 2013	MCH 2012
Effective Pneumonia Care	Pneumonia patients whose initial emergency department blood culture was performed prior to the administration of the hospital dose of antibiotics	97%	98%	99%	98%
Effective Pneumonia Care	Pneumonia patients given the most appropriate initial antibiotics	96%	96%	96%	95%
Timely Surgical Care	Outpatients having surgery who got an antibiotic at the right time (within one hour before surgery)	98%	99%	99%	98%
Timely Surgical Care	Surgery patients who were given an antibiotic at the right time (within one hour before surgery) to help prevent infection	98%	98%	99%	98%
Timely Surgical Care	Surgery patients whose preventive antibiotics were stopped at the right time (within 24 hours after surgery)	97%	96%	97%	98%
Timely Surgical Care	Patients who got treatment at the right time (within 24 hours before or after their surgery) to help prevent blood clot after certain types of surgery.	97%	96%	95%	96%
Effective Surgical Care	Outpatients having surgery who got the right kind of antibiotic	98%	99%	100%	98%

TABLE 5.8
CMS Core Measures for MCH, 2012–2014 (continued)

(continued)

Category	CMS Core Measure	State Benchmark	MCH 2014	MCH 2013	MCH 2012
Effective Surgical Care	Surgery patients who were taking beta blockers before coming to the hospital, who were kept on the beta blockers during the period just before and after the surgery.	96%	94%	93%	90%
Effective Surgical Care	Surgery patients who were given the right kind of antibiotic to help prevent infection	98%	100%	96%	96%
Effective Surgical Care	Heart surgery patients whose blood sugar is kept under good control in the days right after surgery	95%	n/a	n/a	n/a
Effective Surgical Care	Surgery patients whose urinary catheters were removed on the first or second day after surgery	94%	91%	92%	94%
Effective Surgical Care	Patients having surgery who were actively warmed in the operating room or whose body temperature was near normal by the end of surgery	100%	100%	100%	100%
Effective Surgical Care	Surgery patients whose doctor ordered treatments to prevent blood clots after certain types of surgeries	98%	99%	98%	99%
Emergency Department (ED) Care	Average (median) time patient spent in the ED before they were admitted to the hospital as an inpatient (minutes)	Being developed	312	n/a	n/a
Emergency Department (ED) Care	Average (median) time patient spent in the ED, after the doctor decided to admit them as an inpatient before leaving the ED for inpatient care (minutes)	Being developed	186	n/a	n/a

(continued)

Category	CMS Core Measure	State Benchmark	MCH 2014	MCH 2013	MCH 2012
Emergency Department (ED) Care	Average time patients spent in the ED before being sent home (minutes)	Being developed	129	n/a	n/a
Emergency Department (ED) Care	Average time patients who came to the ED with broken bones had to wait before receiving pain medication (minutes)	Being developed	45	n/a	n/a
Emergency Department (ED) Care	Percentage of patients who left the ED before being seen	Being developed	5%	n/a	n/a
Emergency Department (ED) Care	Percentage of patients who came to the emergency department with stoke symptoms who received brain scans results within 45 minutes of arrival	Being developed	n/a	n/a	n/a
Preventive Care	Patients assessed and given influenza vaccination	95%	88%	n/a	n/a
Preventive Care	Patients assessed and given pneumonia vaccination	93%	88%	n/a	n/a
Readmission, Complications, and Death	Rate of readmission for heart attack	No different from US national rate			
Readmission, Complications, and Death	Death rate for heart attack patients	No different from US national rate			
Readmission, Complications, and Death	Rate of Readmission for heart failure patients	No different from US national rate			
Readmission, Complications, and Death	Rate of readmission for pneumonia patients	No different from US national rate			

TABLE 5.8
CMS Core Measures for MCH, 2012–2014 (continued)

(continued)

Category	CMS Core Measure	State Benchmark	MCH 2014	MCH 2013	MCH 2012
Serious Complications and Deaths	Serious complications - rate	No different from US national rate			
Hospital-Acquired Conditions	Hospital-acquired conditions	Being developed	n/a	n/a	n/a
Healthcare-Associated Infections	Central line–associated bloodstream infections	No different from the US national benchmark			
Use of Medical Imaging	Outpatients with low back pain who had an MRI without trying recommended treatments first, such as PT	32.9%	29%	28%	34%
Use of Medical Imaging	Outpatients who had a follow-up mammogram or ultrasound within 45 days after a screening mammogram	12.4%	12%	12%	9%
Use of Medical Imaging	Outpatient CT scans of the chest that were "combination" scans	0.03%	Less than 1%	Less than 1%	Less than 1%
Use of Medical Imaging	Outpatient CT scans of the abdomen that were "combination" scans	0.07%	Less than 1%	Less than 1%	Less than 1%
Use of Medical Imaging	Outpatients who got cardiac imaging stress tests before low-risk outpatient surgery	Being developed	8%	9%	7%
Use of Medical Imaging	Outpatients with brain CT scans who got a sinus CT scan at the same time	Being developed	5%	7%	5%
Patient Survey Results	Patients who reported that their nurses "always" communicated well	84%	72%	60%	80%
Patient Survey Results	Patients who reported that their doctor "always" communicated well	80%	74%	77%	71%

(continued)

Category	CMS Core Measure	State Benchmark	MCH 2014	MCH 2013	MCH 2012
Patient Survey Results	Patients who reported they "always" received help as soon as they wanted	62%	58%	59%	60%
Patient Survey Results	Patients who reported that their pain was "always" well controlled	75%	70%	63%	70%
Patient Survey Results	Patients who reported that staff "always" explained about medicine before giving it to them	69%	74%	64%	70%
Patient Survey Results	Patients who reported that their room and bathroom were "always" clean	73%	82%	84%	80%
Patient Survey Results	Patients who reported that the area around their room was "always" quiet at night	73%	50%	52%	50%
Patient Survey Results	Patients at each hospital who reported "yes," they were given information about what to do during their recovery at home	85%	94%	98%	93%
Patient Survey Results	Patients who gave their hospital a rating of 9 or 10 on a scale from 0 to 10	68%	61%	62%	60%
Patient Survey Results	Patients who reported "yes," they would definitely recommend the hospital	76%	80%	75%	76%

TABLE 5.8
CMS Core Measures for MCH, 2012–2014 (continued)

NOTES: "n/a" means not applicable and that the data are either not available or that the number of cases is too small for a legitimate conclusion. "Being developed" means that the core measure remains under development and no standard or benchmark has yet to be published. "State" means the statewide mean score.

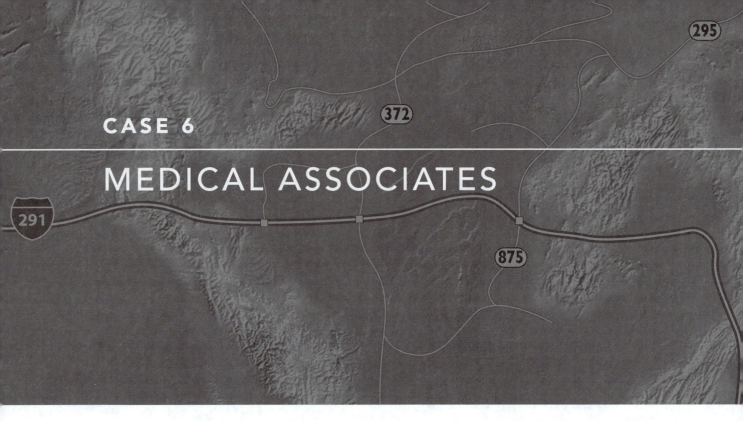

MEDICAL ASSOCIATES

Medical Associates is a for-profit medical group of 40 physicians. It operates two facilities—one in Middleboro, approximately three miles from Middleboro Community Hospital, and one in Jasper, on the eastern edge of Jasper. Each facility is a modern one-story building with ample parking and room for expansion. The Middleboro facility opened in 1995. The facility in Jasper opened in 2002.

Medical Associates currently provides services in the following medical specialties:

- Cardiology

- ENT

- Family medicine

- Gastroenterology

- General surgery

- Internal medicine

- OB/GYN

- Orthopedic surgery

◆   Pediatrics

◆   Urology

All physicians maintain active medical staff privileges at an accredited hospital and consulting staff privileges at other appropriate hospitals. Currently, 23 physicians staff the facility in Middleboro. Many maintain active medical privileges at Middleboro Community Hospital. Many also maintain consulting staff privileges at Capital City General Hospital. In Jasper, 17 Medical Associates physicians provide medical services. Of these 17, some maintain medical privileges at Middleboro Community Hospital. The others maintain active staff privileges at Capital City General Hospital and consulting staff medical privileges at Middleboro Community Hospital. Some only maintain privileges at other hospitals located in Capital City and Middleboro.

At each facility Medical Associates maintains a drawing station for Wythe Laboratories, Inc., of Capital City. Comprehensive imaging services including ultrasound, radiographic, CT and MRI technologies are also available in each location. Ambulatory surgical services, begun in January 2014, are available on site at the Jasper facility.

HISTORY

Founded in 1951, Medical Associates was originally a single-specialty medical practice. Under the leadership of Dr. James R. Fairchild, a board-certified internist, it slowly expanded in size and in 1963 began to add other specialties. Since 1972, it has provided specialty and subspecialty medical and surgical care.

Dr. Fairchild was an early proponent of multispecialty medical care. For almost 15 years, he chaired the committee on multispecialty medical practice of the State Medical Society. Twice he received special awards from the American Medical Association for articles he wrote that examined the value of multispecialty medicine in rural areas. For many years he personally recruited all new physicians.

Trained in internal medicine at a midwestern medical school, Dr. Fairchild completed his residency training at a large midwestern medical center known for its innovative approaches to serving rural areas using a large multispecialty group. As he later expressed in his articles and many speeches, he advocated multispecialty medical practices as "medical practices that truly serve the patient's interests of high quality, convenience, and reasonable costs." In 1972, under his leadership, Medical Associates required "all affiliated physicians to be board certified within three years." At that time, this decision was considered to be controversial. Throughout his career with Medical Associates, Dr. Fairchild has served as its president and medical director. Until 1972, when a full-time executive manager was added, Dr. Fairchild also supervised all professional and administrative staff. On the occasion of Dr. Fairchild's retirement from Medical Associates, the facility in Jasper was renamed the

Fairchild Medical Center. Dr. Fairchild is retired but still attends most board meetings as an "interested observer."

Dr. Fairchild, however, was a significant long-term critic of the hospitals located in Middleboro. When he retired in 1988, he blamed "the lack of innovation in medical care in our communities on the self-interested behaviors and approaches each hospital has followed for decades." According to Fairchild, "The problem in our community is our hospitals—they do not listen to the practicing physician who knows best the needs of patients." In 1972, Medical Associates hired its first physician trained in osteopathic medicine (DO), an individual who subsequently became a partner in Medical Associates. This physician practiced in Jasper using the hospital resources in Capital City. According to Dr. Fairchild, Dr. Maynard Krebs was "one of our finest primary care physicians before primary care became the rage; he practiced successfully with Medical Associates for many years and even has a memorial dedicated to him and his services at Osteopathic General Hospital in Capital City."

Over the past 15 years, all of the original physicians affiliated with Medical Associates have either retired or left the area. Many new physicians have joined Medical Associates in the past ten years, most coming to Medical Associates immediately after completing a residency in their medical specialty.

GOVERNANCE AND ORGANIZATION

Medical Associates is organized as a for-profit, professional corporation. Each shareholder in the corporation has rights to distributed earnings based upon a predetermined formula approved by the board of directors. The total number of Medical Associates shares equals the number of shareholder physicians. New physicians are recruited and hired on a two-year contract that provides a fixed salary and benefits. At the end of two years, the new physician is either offered the opportunity to join Medical Associates as a shareholder or is terminated. If offered the opportunity to join Medical Associates as a shareholder, the physician must purchase from Medical Associates one share in the practice. When a physician leaves Medical Associates, Medical Associates repurchases her share of stock. The bylaws of the corporation establish the methodology for this rate of buy-in and severance. The rate is "equal to the total equity of the corporation divided by the number of partner physicians." The bylaws also establish that this methodology can be changed by a two-thirds vote of the partner physicians.

Each physician affiliated with Medical Associates has signed a contractual covenant that, should he or the group terminate his relationship with Medical Associates, he cannot practice within a 30-mile radius of Middleboro for two years without paying compensatory damages equal to the compensation he received from the group for the previous two years. In 1978, this covenant was tested in state court and found to be legal. Since that time, no former Medical Associate physician has disputed this covenant.

ORGANIZATION OF THE BOARD OF DIRECTORS

A seven-member elected board of directors represents shareholder interests. Each director serves a three-year term. Terms are staggered so that no more than three new directors are elected annually. No term limits exist. The full board meets monthly and hosts its annual meeting in December, during which the board members whose terms are not expiring elect new directors, with each shareholder having one vote. All shareholders are invited to the annual meeting. Continuing board members serve as a nominating committee and formally recommend a slate of candidates. New board members take office on January 1 of the following year. Once the new board members have been elected, the entire new board then elects its president, vice president, secretary, and treasurer.

Between monthly meetings, standing committees meet. Any five board members can request a special meeting of the board by providing written notice to the president.

Membership of the Board of Directors, as of January 1, 2014

Name	Department	Term Expires	Board Position
R. Samuels	Pediatrics	2016	President
J. Putter	Surgery, general	2017	Vice president
K. Kipstein	Cardiology	2015	Secretary
D. Fixer	Urology	2016	Treasurer
M. Stanley	Surgery, orthopedic	2017	At large
S. Lee	Surgery, orthopedic	2016	At large
U. Unvey	Pediatrics	2015	At large

The board has four standing committees and uses ad hoc committees as needed. Standing committees make recommendations to the full board. Standing committees include the following:

AUDIT COMMITTEE

This committee is chaired by the board's treasurer and is composed of two other board members. It oversees the preparation for Medical Associate's annual financial audit by an independent accounting firm. It is responsible for implementing all recommendations in the auditor's management letter. Every three years the committee recommends to the board who should perform the audit. Current members of this committee are Dr. Douglas Fixer (chair), Dr. Mark Stanley, and Walter Graham (ex officio).

CLINICAL STANDARDS AND QUALITY

This committee is chaired by the board's vice president and includes one other board member and the medical director (ex officio, unless also an elected member of the board). This committee annually reviews the group's medical quality assurance plan and systems to monitor and manage quality. It also reviews the medical credentials of any new physician. Every third year, it recommends to the board who should be appointed (or reappointed) as medical director. Currently this committee oversees the meaningful use program that launched in 2012. This committee also addresses all questions concerning the credentials and fitness of physicians. Current members of this committee are Dr. Jules Putter (chair), Dr. Ursula Unvey, and Dr. Clyde Eason (ex officio, medical director).

FINANCE COMMITTEE

This committee meets monthly to review the organization's financial statements and make recommendations to the full board. It also reviews the budget recommended by the executive manager and recommends this budget to the board for ratification. Medical Associates' fiscal year begins on January 1 and ends on December 31. In the December meeting the board generally approves the budget for an upcoming fiscal year. Current members of this committee are Dr. Kevin Kipstein (chair), Dr. Sarah Lee, and Graham (ex officio).

MANAGEMENT COMMITTEE

The board's president chairs this committee. Other members include the medical director, the chair of each medical department, one other board member, and the executive manager. This committee meets monthly to review the operations, including the budget performance, and to address management problems and issues. Current members of this committee are Robert Samuels (president and chair), Dr. Kipstein, Dr. Eason (medical director), Dr. Putter (chair of surgery), Thomas Underwood (chair of medicine), and Graham (executive manager).

MEDICAL DEPARTMENTS AND ORGANIZATION

Medical Associates' medical director is appointed for a three-year term by the board. Medical Associates has two medical departments: primary care and surgery. In accordance with the organization's bylaws, "the medical director cannot be the board's president or vice president." The medical director oversees the development and implementation of the medical quality assurance plan, medical care protocols, and (with participating insurance plans) the formulary. The medical director must approve all new or revised contracts involving ancillary services, such as imaging and laboratory services, before the president can sign the contract. Increasingly, the medical director is responsible for all relations and contracts with managed care plans. As compensation, the medical director receives an extra 15 percent of his practice-based compensation.

Each department chair is elected annually in December by the physician shareholders assigned to the specific medical department. The chair receives an extra 12 percent stipend in addition to any practice-based compensation. A chair is responsible for convening monthly medical staff meetings and representing the medical department on the management committee. Each chair also serves as the supervisor for all professional and administrative staff assigned to the medical department, such as registered nurses, medical assistants, and receptionists.

Dr. Eason is the current medical director. He has held this position for the past seven years. Dr. Eason is a graduate of an eastern medical school and completed advanced education in his medical specialty at a major midwestern medical center. He also holds a master's of public health in occupational medicine. He is board certified in both his internal medicine subspecialty and occupational health. Born in the area, Dr. Eason returned upon completion of his medical education. He has been associated with Medical Associates for 15 years. He is married to a member of the Fairchild family.

Dr. Putter is the chief of the department of surgery. He has held this position for the past seven years. Dr. Putter is a graduate of a western medical school and completed a degree in advanced medical education in general surgery at a major midwestern teaching hospital. Medical Associates recruited him 20 years ago. On three previous occasions, Dr. Putter has served on the board of directors of Medical Associates. On two of these occasions, he served as president.

Dr. Underwood is chief of the department of medicine. He was recently elected to this position for the first time. Dr. Underwood is a graduate of a southern medical school and completed his advanced medical education at teaching hospitals located in both the Midwest and East. Dr. Underwood previously served as chair of the board's ad hoc committee on long range planning and medical recruitment.

The chief of a medical department determines physician work schedules. The medical director resolves any disputes. All physicians rotate Saturdays and on-call duties. In the past, physicians typically worked one Saturday every six weeks.

ADMINISTRATIVE AND OTHER SERVICES

Medical Associates employs a full-time executive manager, Walter Graham, responsible for patient accounts, communications, building maintenance and grounds, materials management, medical records, information systems, imaging, laboratory services, and all nonclinical staff. He also serves as the controller for the corporation. He reports directly to the president. Graham is a graduate of State University and holds a graduate degree in health services administration from a western university. He has been an active member of the Medical Group Management Association for the past 20 years and has served in various administrative capacities in multispecialty medical groups for the past 28 years. Medical Associates has employed him for six years because of his extensive background in medical group management. He has worked with the board to enhance the appointment and electronic medical records systems and to install new information systems for accounting and medical information.

Graham maintains an office in the Middleboro facility and travels to Jasper at least once a week. All employees not assigned to a specific physician or to ambulatory surgery (e.g., registered nurses, medical assistants) also report directly to him, including Ellen Smythe (head of patient accounts and business operations), Steve Mangrove (bookkeeper), Hank Hammer (maintenance chief), Mary Folder (head of medical records), Alice Byte (director for information systems), Mary Kitchen (imaging services, Middleboro), Warren Kidder (imaging services, Jasper), Robin Swisher (laboratory services, Middleboro), and Helen Morgan (laboratory services, Jasper).

The Middleboro facility has a centralized appointment system and patient registration service as well as a waiting area. Physician suites (each with two or three examination rooms) are assigned by medical specialty. Currently, family medicine and pediatrics are located in the east and west wing, and surgery is located in the south wing. The center of the facility houses the common waiting area and patient accounts. All other departments are located in the basement. The Jasper facility also has a centralized appointment system and patient registration service and waiting area. Currently, family medicine and pediatrics are located in the front wing while surgery is located in the rear wing with medical records, imaging, and laboratory. All physician suites have three examination rooms.

At the Jasper facility, medical records, imaging, and laboratory are each part of their counterpart department in the Middleboro facility. All other services (e.g., patient accounts) are provided directly through the Middleboro facility using telecommunications and computer systems. On January 15, 2014, Medical Associates opened an ambulatory surgical facility in the basement area of the Jasper facility. Ambulatory surgery services are provided five days per week, with most surgeries scheduled between 7:30 a.m. and 3:00 p.m. Two fully equipped surgical suites are available. The area also includes a modern waiting and recovery area. Mary Knoph, RN, is the director of this facility. She reports to the chief of the department of surgery.

Medical Associates contracts with Wythe Laboratories in Capital City for medical tests. In-house laboratory services are limited to blood chemistries and urine analyses done using equipment leased and calibrated by Wythe Laboratories. Medical Associates also contracts with Radiology Partners in Capital City to read all diagnostic images. Under a newly installed system, radiographic and MRI and CT images are transmitted electronically to this group, which reads and files a report electronically. Under the existing agreement, Medical Associates owns and operates its own imaging equipment and employs the needed technicians. Ultrasound imaging is also available in both locations. Radiology Partners is only responsible for reading and interpreting medical images. Other contracted services at both locations include snow removal and grounds maintenance, custodial services, and laundry services.

When asked to describe his most significant accomplishments over the past three years, Graham said that as a result of careful investments Medical Associates has a state-of-the-art electronic health record that could—if desired—be linked to the electronic medical record systems of any of the area hospitals. He indicated that defining this system, getting board approval for the systems, and then overseeing its installation and field-testing was the most complex project he undertook in his career. Other points he raised included the new appointment system and the (slow) progress associated with the better management of accounts receivable and payable. He stated that the Middleboro facility is ready for the introduction of ambulatory surgery as soon as the board authorizes it. "I am also very satisfied with the national consulting firm that is helping us under the federal meaningful use program. We are seeing some changes in clinical practice and continue to qualify for the maximum federal benefits."

PHYSICAL FACILITIES

In Middleboro, Medical Associates occupies a modern 48,500-square-foot, T-shaped, one-story building with ample parking and room for expansion. The building was opened in 1995 and modernized and expanded in 2002. The building is organized into four areas with a total of 25 medical suites. It was last renovated in 2006. In 2007 this facility was highlighted in the periodical *Medical Group News*.

Medical Associates' Jasper facility is located in a modern one-story, 42,590-square-foot, H-shaped building built in 2002. The facility has 20 medical suites and ample parking. When the land was originally purchased in 1990, Medical Associates also acquired a 30-year option on a 225-acre undeveloped parcel adjacent to this facility, an action Dr. Fairchild had to lobby for before it was finally approved. This option, which cost $35,000, establishes a purchase price not to exceed "the average prevailing rate plus 10 percent for undeveloped farm land in Hillsboro County as established by independent appraisal." Medical Associates has been contacted within the past six months to determine whether it would sell or execute this land option. The land is adjacent to the newly approved highway's Jasper interchange.

Recently Medical Associates and Cardiology Hospitals of America (CHA) announced a joint feasibility project to build and construct a cardiac hospital in Jasper to service Hillsboro County and surrounding areas. Under the feasibility agreement, Medical

Associates would have the ability to financially participate in this project and be a significant (but minority) owner in this proprietary hospital. In announcing this study, Dr. Herman Goodfellow, president of CHA, stated that this project should have little or no discernable impact on neighboring general hospitals. "CHA hospitals bring the newest technologies to a community—technologies that general hospitals may not be able to afford or support; our number one goal is to address heart disease. We don't have a number two goal." A formal feasibility report is expected within three months. The Jasper Industrial Development Authority estimates that this new hospital could be a top-ten employer within five years of opening and has tentatively agreed to lease this hospital land in the Jasper Industrial Park. The authority also indicated that this new hospital would generate a significant amount of tax revenue. Dr. Goodfellow stated in his press briefing that this hospital will serve residents from throughout Hillsboro County, as well as from Capital City and University Town, and that the new hospital will invite appropriate affiliations with physicians located in these areas.

Dr. Samuels, president of Medical Associates, said that Medical Associates could either donate or lease land for the project and that it would want all physicians affiliated with this hospital to be affiliated with Medical Associates. He also indicated the challenges associated with the existing Certificate of Need (CON) law and regulations but felt that collaboratively Medical Associates and CHA could secure either a legislative or gubernatorial special exemption. Another option might be to be ready to undertake this project if and when the CON law lapses. Dr. Samuels has requested that the State Medical Society advocate that CON lapse as scheduled.

OPERATIONS

Medical Associates in open six days per week in each location from 8:00 a.m. until 6:00 p.m. Medical Associates is closed Sundays and on all federal holidays. When it is closed, all telephone inquiries before midnight are handled by a registered nurse. After midnight but before 8:00 am, inquiries are handled by an answering service, which contacts on-call physicians as needed. Beginning in late 2015, Medical Associates will extend its hours to 9:00 p.m. on two evening per week. Detailed plans of how this will be accomplished are currently being developed.

All full-time employees work a 40-hour week and qualify for a full benefit package that includes two weeks' vacation and family coverage in a comprehensive health and dental insurance plan. Sick days are earned by employees at the rate of one per month, with a maximum bank of thirty days. Medical Associates maintains a 401(k) retirement plan for all employees but does not contribute as part of any benefit plan. Part-time employees are hired at an hourly rate and receive no voluntary benefits or vacation. Any part-time employee who is scheduled to work more than 948 hours in a calendar year may purchase the health insurance plan through Medical Associates by paying the prorated difference between the percentage of time worked and the total annual premium.

All physicians are also provided comprehensive benefits, including full payment of medical liability insurance and five days for continuing medical education. Staff physicians are hired for a fixed two-year salary negotiated at the time of their appointment and qualify for four weeks of paid vacation per year.

Shareholding physicians are compensated using a predetermined formula based on the revenue (the net revenue Medical Associates receives for the services provided by the physician) they generate offset by their expenses (the physician's share of all direct and indirect costs associated with her practice). During the fiscal year, each physician is compensated monthly based on an estimated difference between revenue and expenses. At the end of the fiscal year, the physician is provided the total difference between total funds previously drawn and her total share of corporate earnings as determined by the formula. To qualify for 100 percent of her share, the physician must work 230 days in a fiscal year. The total draw is reduced on a straight percentage basis for each day under the 230 days. Physicians who work more than 230 days share on a pro rata basis.

INSURANCE AND REIMBURSEMENT

Medical Associates provides services on a fee-for-service basis. Medical Associates has a long-standing policy of accepting "any insurance plan presented to us by one of our patients." As such, Medical Associates has a contractual relationship with area preferred provider organizations (PPOs) including Blue Shield, the Central States Good Health Network, and two commercial PPOs. Medical Associates also maintains a contractual relationship with managed care plans offered by Blue Shield and commercial providers.

Three years ago, Medical Associates accepted an exclusive contractual relationship with Swift Health Plan, a statewide HMO, to provide services to the plan's members. This contract will lapse within six months. Medical Associates is the only medical provider under this HMO in Middleboro and Mifflenville.

Prices charged at both facilities are exactly the same. All patients are provided a detailed bill or account statement. For patients covered by Blue Shield (indemnity), Medical Associates directly bills Blue Shield and then bills the patient for any outstanding balances. Patients covered by other forms of indemnity insurance are required to pay (cash, check, or credit card) and are provided a bill to send to their insurance carrier for reimbursement. These independent corporations bill separately for laboratory services provided by Wythe Laboratories and reading services done by Radiology Partners.

Medical Associates generally discounts its listed fees by 3 percent on its managed care contracts, excluding the contact with the Swift Health Plan, which receives a 7 percent discount. The basic visit fee is $125.

Medicare accounts for approximately 35 percent of Medical Associates' total gross revenue, and Medicaid accounts for approximately 15 percent. The other 50 percent of total gross revenue comes primarily from insurance.

CURRENT ISSUES

LAND OPTION

The 30-year option on the parcel adjacent to the Jasper facility establishes a purchase price not to exceed "the average prevailing rate plus 10 percent for undeveloped farm land in Hillsboro County." Currently, this average prevailing rate is $2,800 per acre, and it is expected to increase. Any undeveloped land the organization acquires will be taxed at the rate of $500 per acre per year with a 5 percent increase per year. The 225-acre parcel, once acquired, could immediately be subdivided. The 25 acres adjacent to the anticipated new highway could be sold for $20,000 per acre. The remaining land would then be owned and retained by Medical Associates for potential expansion or subsequent sale, or it could be sold for prevailing rate. A local real estate developer has indicated that his corporation would buy the entire parcel for $1 million. Medical Associates has been advised that any financial action it takes should not raise its long-term debt to net asset ratio higher than 27.5 percent. The hurdle rate is 6 percent, and the organization can borrow funds at 3.5 percent. Medical Associates needs to develop a business plan regarding this land option.

AMBULATORY SURGERY FOR MIDDLEBORO

Medical Associates has achieved its first-year targeted utilization and financial projections for ambulatory surgery in Jasper. It is now time to consider a similar service at the Middleboro facility. The physical facilities needed for ambulatory surgery will cost approximately $750,000 for renovation and expansion, with approximately $350,000 of that estimated for needed equipment. Current area prices are approximately $100 per square foot for renovation and $250 per square foot for new construction.

The basement of the Middleboro facility has sufficient space for ambulatory surgery similar to the facility created at the Jasper office. Existing mechanical systems and parking are sufficient to support this new service.

Medical Associates faces a 3.5 percent cost of capital. The anticipated salvage value of these new fixed assets will be $350,000 after five years. To do this project Medical Associates needs to recruit at least one or two new general surgeons or ENT physicians for the Jasper office, thereby freeing the Middleboro physicians to work in this new ambulatory surgical facility. Based on preliminary estimates, the organization anticipates that this project's operational revenue will exceed total expenses for each of the first five years. Medical Associates estimates that this unit, using the standard RVU system used in hospitals, will generate 1.1 surgical procedures per case.

MEDICAL APPOINTMENT SYSTEMS—PEDIATRICS AND OB/GYN

National studies suggest that, on average, pediatricians devote 92 percent of their time to ambulatory appointments and OB/GYN physicians devote 70 percent. Currently, the appointment system uses 15-minute appointments in pediatrics (four per hour) and 20 minutes in OB/GYN (three per hour). The mean service rate as determined by a special study is 5.0 per hour in pediatrics and 4.5 per hour in OB/GYN. Medical Associates is concerned that demand will quickly outpace its ability to serve these patients and needs an independent review of its current systems and capacities.

REGISTERED NURSES VERSUS MEDICAL ASSISTANTS

Five years ago, Medical Associates began to change its staffing from relying solely upon registered nurses (RNs) to hiring medical assistants (MAs). Currently all physicians assigned to primary care service are assigned one RN or MA to assist with patient care. Physicians assigned to surgery are assigned one RN for every two physicians. As RNs retire or resign, they have been replaced with MAs. On five recent occasions, when an RN assigned to a senior physician resigned, the senior physician demanded that the RN assigned to a staff physician (nonshareholder) be reassigned to him and that a new MA be hired to fill the vacancy with the staff physician.

This ad hoc system of job switching has caused internal turmoil between the senior and junior physicians and has led to the subsequent resignation of two RNs who did not want to be reassigned. In 2010, one staff physician resigned from Medical Associates and cited this as the primary reason for deciding to relocate his practice. Trying to resolve this issue has led to many discussions. Confusion exists around staff reporting relationships and who has the authority to change job assignments. Some believe that staff reports to the physician for whom they actually work. Others say the authority lies with the chief of the medical department, administration, or the board of directors. At the last three board meetings, this issue has been discussed with no resolution. Dr. Doris Dustin has recently filed a formal complaint with the board concerning the upcoming reassignment of her nurse to Dr. Quinton Reeper in pediatrics.

INTERNAL ORGANIZATION, MANAGEMENT, AND SYSTEMS IMPROVEMENT

Graham has recently recommended that Medical Associates recruit and hire a deputy executive manager for human resources. His rationale is that "this portion of my position has grown and continued to take valuable time away from my other duties, including being the comptroller for the corporation." Graham has stated that his job responsibilities, including attending all board and board committee meetings, "exceed my ability to function effectively." On discussion with Graham, management agreed that an outside consultant would review the internal organization and management of Medical Associates.

Graham did indicate when discussing human resource issues and challenges that similar medical groups directly assign all nonphysician personnel to be supervised by the executive manager. Physicians generally do not supervise any staff. Graham said he is prepared to become the supervisor for all nonphysicians. Note that at least two members of the board believe that "we spend too much on administration already."

OTHER ISSUES

Graham also mentioned that he believes that his annual salary of $105,000 is significantly below market.

FINANCIAL STRUCTURE

Another issue of long-term concern for Medical Associates involves the financial structure of the corporation. At a recent board retreat, a consultant recommended that the corporation retain more of its annual earnings before sharing them with the shareholders. He specifically recommended that the overhead cost be increased to include at least an additional 6 percent contribution to net assets. This report was controversial. Some physicians want to avoid being taxed twice, first on corporate profits and then on individual income. As one physician noted, "If we don't make a large corporate profit, we minimize our corporate taxes."

AREA HMOS

Dr. Eason, the medical director, recently informed the board of his growing concern over managed care practices in the area. Increasingly, closed-panel HMOs are attempting to mandate the medical practice of physicians retained outside the panel and want to hold the physician (or medical group) responsible for any costs associated with deviations from HMO-approved practice patterns.

For the past seven years, Medical Associates physicians have been retained by Swift Health Plan, a closed-panel HMO, to provide services to subscribers in their area. Recently, Swift informed Dr. Eason that, unless Medical Associates physicians adhered to "approved practice protocols," Swift would have to terminate its relationship with Medical Associates and "employ its own physicians in this area."

While Dr. Eason has identified this issue as important, he has offered no solution. The Medical Appointment and Practices Committee of the board has recently reviewed the cases being questioned by Swift and found that "in every instance, we conclude that our physician acted in the best interests of his or her patient."

Dr. Eason also informed all the physicians in Medical Associates that they need to "come to agreement" on the issue of "exclusivity and HMOs." As he expressed it, "It is simple. Are we willing to sign a contract with a specific HMO that requires us to forgo opportunities with other HMOs?" He reported on two occasions being approached by HMOs from Capital City who are interested in Jasper. Each indicated that, if Medical Associates did not sign an exclusive contract with them, they just "might" put some primary care physicians in Jasper and start referring even more patients to their physicians in Capital City when the patients need hospital-based services. Dr. Eason has identified exclusivity as the most important issue the board needs to resolve within the next 12 to 18 months.

OTHER CONCERNS

The clinical standards and quality committee recently recommended that at least two additional primary care physicians be added to the Jasper facility. This recommendation has (again) opened the issue of whether Medical Associates should recruit physicians trained in family practice as opposed to physicians trained in general internal medicine, OB/GYN, or pediatrics. Dr. Putter, chief of surgery and chair of this committee, recently submitted a compelling argument in favor of family practice physicians to this committee only to be directly challenged by Dr. Underwood. Dr. Putter has indicated that his committee remains gridlocked on this issue and cannot proceed with any recruiting until it is resolved.

This committee has also reported to the board that Medical Associates needs one or two professional staff analysts if it is to fulfill the expectations associated with medical outcome studies that HMO clients and Blue Shield have requested. Dr. Eason has informed the board that he currently devotes approximately 20 percent of his time to requests for this type of information and that he needs professional assistance to relieve him of this burden. The board has yet to act upon his request. The budget for 2015, however, was approved without the staff previously requested by Dr. Eason.

Graham's three-year contract expires at the end of 2015. Unless this contract is renegotiated by July 1, 2015, Graham has the contractual option to elect his one-year's severance pay. Dr. Stanley (at his first board meeting) was surprised to learn that no job description existed for the executive manager's position. He asked at that time, "Without a job description, how can appropriate compensation be determined?" In reply, Dr. Samuels informed him, "Everyone knows what Walter does. Why do we need to waste another sheet of paper on this, too?"

Medical referrals have always occurred within Medical Associates. Patients are referred to another Medical Associates physician as warranted by the patient's need. The opening of the new ambulatory surgical service in the Jasper facility, however, is beginning to stress the surgeons from Middleboro. Surgeons based at the Middleboro office are now expected to perform certain outpatient surgeries in Jasper. As stated by Dr. Harvey Hersh, a general surgeon in the Middleboro facility, "I am beginning to spend too much 'windshield' time traveling back and forth between our two facilities and seeing my patients in the hospital. Something needs to be done. My time is too valuable to spend it in my car." Dr. Eason has met with the surgeons and has explained that a certain level of inconvenience is necessary in the short run until this new service is established. The Middleboro surgeons accepted Dr. Eason's promise that this problem would be corrected in the next three to six months.

Jeffrey Whittier, regional vice president of Clearwater Medical Systems, a publicly traded corporation that owns and operates physician offices and groups, has recently contacted Medical Associates to determine whether it is for sale. Whittier indicated that Clearwater would be "interested in furnishing an offer if Medical Associates would seriously consider it." Dr. Samuels has indicated that Medical Associates will reply to his inquiry after the next meeting of the board.

OHA Ventures of Capital City has also expressed interest in Medical Associates and said it would like the opportunity to develop a proposal for either the outright purchase of Medical Associates in Jasper or the purchase of the Jasper facility, which would then be leased back to Medical Associates at a specific long-term rate.

At the last board meeting the board instructed Dr. Eason to secure additional consultants to help the board to develop an appropriate strategy for responding to the creation of accountable care organizations and changes in the federal Patient Protection and Affordable Care Act.

Additional information regarding Medical Associates' staffing, utilization, compensation, financial status, and operations may be found in the following tables.

TABLE 6.1
Physicians Affiliated with Medical Associates as of December 31, 2014

Name	Specialty	Age	Office	Active	Consulting
Autumn	Gastroenterology	44	Middleboro	MCH	CCG
Barton	Internal medicine	45	Middleboro	MCH	CCG
Coolidge	ENT	44	Jasper	CGS	OMC, WH
Douglas	Internal medicine	41	Middleboro	MCH	CCG
Dustin	OB/GYN	33	Middleboro	MCH	CCG
Eason	Urology	56	Middleboro	MCH	CCG
Finn	Surgery	47	Jasper	CCG	MCH
Fixer	Urology	43	Middleboro	MCH	CCG
Frost	Internal medicine	41	Jasper	MCH	CGS
Goldwater	Orthopedic surgery	44	Jasper	CGS	WH, OMC
Gost	OB/GYN	45	Middleboro	MCH	CCG
Hersh	General surgery	40	Middleboro	MCH	CCG
Jackson	General surgery	39	Middleboro	MCH	CCG
Kessler	Internal medicine	34	Middleboro	MCH	CCG
Kipstein	Cardiology	50	Jasper	CGS	MGH
Klock	OB/GYN	49	Jasper	CGS	MGH
Lee	Orthopedic surgery	40	Jasper	CGS	MGH
Lesko	Internal medicine	38	Middleboro	MCH	CCG
Maeer	Cardiology	42	Jasper	CGS	MGH
Master	Internal medicine	40	Middleboro	MCH	CCG
Chan	Pediatrics	37	Jasper	CGS	MGH
Mustard	OB/GYN	39	Jasper	CGS	MGH
Never	General surgery	45	Middleboro	MCH	CCG
O'Connell	General surgery	49	Middleboro	MCH	CCG
Otter	Pediatrics	37	Jasper	CGS	MGH
Picture	Orthopedic surgery	47	Jasper	CGS	MGH
Polk	OB/GYN	40	Jasper	OMC	WH
Putter	General surgery	62	Middleboro	MCH	CCG

(continued)

TABLE 6.1

Physicians
Affiliated with
Medical Associates
as of December
31, 2014
(continued)

Name	Specialty	Age	Office	Active	Consulting
Qestrom	Orthopedic surgery	39	Middleboro	MCH	CCG
Quester	Pediatrics	40	Jasper	MCH	CGS
Reeper	Pediatrics	59	Middleboro	MCH	CCG
Samuels	Pediatrics	47	Middleboro	MCH	CCG
St. James	Pediatrics	40	Middleboro	MCH	CCG
Stanley	Orthopedic surgery	49	Middleboro	MCH	CCG
Steve	Orthopedic surgery	47	Jasper	CGS	MCH
Underwood	Cardiology	46	Middleboro	MCH	CCG
Unvey	Pediatrics	56	Jasper	MCH	CGS
Washington	Internal medicine	43	Jasper	CCG	WH
Weckensen	ENT	44	Middleboro	MCH	CCG
Xerox	ENT	42	Middleboro	MCH	CCG

NOTES: Active = Active medical staff privileges by hospital

Consulting = Consulting medical staff privileges by hospital

MCH = Middleboro Community Hospital

WH = Webster Hospital

CCG = Capital City General

OMC= Osteopathic Medical Center, Capital City

(This table can also be found online at ache.org/books/Middleboro.)

Name	Specialty	2014			2013			2012		
		APPTS	P-Days	DIS	APPTS	P-Days	DIS	APPTS	P-Days	DIS
Department of Primary Care										
S. St. James	Pediatrics	5,521	120	45	5,432	135	40	5,234	178	59
R. Samuels	Pediatrics	5,167	114	29	5,234	123	30	5,005	126	32
Q. Reeper	Pediatrics	5,234	99	25	5,134	102	24	4,687	98	32
G. Gost	OB/GYN	4,319	720	177	4,138	734	164	4,023	793	170
D. Dustin	OB/GYN	4,625	650	193	4,456	645	187	4,044	696	190
Z. Autumn	Gastroenterology	2,789	755	156	2,705	745	144	2,656	801	131
W. Xerox	ENT	2,845	504	131	2,840	512	134	3,405	529	143
V. Weckensen	ENT	2,945	483	104	2,834	477	99	2,341	490	105
T. Underwood	Cardiology	4,456	677	133	4,178	606	105	4,277	545	109
D. Fixer	Urology	2,403	578	143	2,202	598	142	2,005	612	157
C. Eason	Urology	1,645	457	101	1,470	459	101	1,034	499	101
M. Master	Internal medicine	3,623	492	102	4,263	501	102	2,330	535	135
L. Lesko	Internal medicine	4,034	560	102	4,083	525	98	4,405	555	99
K. Kessler*	Internal medicine	4,256	712	161	2,033	204	45	0	0	0
C. Douglas	Internal medicine	4,340	820	210	4,256	834	187	4,456	902	167
A. Barton	Internal medicine	4,206	850	177	4,256	654	152	4,124	756	165
	Subtotals	**62,408**	**8,591**	**1,989**	**59,514**	**7,854**	**1,754**	**54,026**	**8,115**	**1,795**
Department of Surgery										
H. Never	General	2,546	870	215	2,206	830	204	2,345	854	207
J. Putter	General	912	630	126	1,112	720	160	1,345	779	199
L. O'Connell	General	1,456	416	104	1,045	418	103	867	436	109
D. Jackson	General	1,843	792	167	1,678	722	134	1,767	812	99
B. Hersh	General	1,245	1,200	267	1,045	1,103	245	1,956	1,223	265
M. Stanley	Orthopedic	1,766	1,544	279	1,862	1,647	298	2,645	1,767	202
K. Qestrom	Orthopedic	1,799	1,433	220	1,566	1,153	208	2,675	1,254	267
	Subtotals	**11,567**	**6,885**	**1,378**	**10,514**	**6,593**	**1,352**	**13,600**	**7,125**	**1,348**
	Total	**73,975**	**15,476**	**3,367**	**70,028**	**14,447**	**3,106**	**67,626**	**15,240**	**3,143**

TABLE 6.2

Utilization Statistics—Middleboro Office

NOTES: APPTS = Appointments
P-Days - Patient days (all hospitals)
DIS = Discharges (all hospitals)
* = Hired July 1, 2013

(This table can also be found online at ache.org/books/Middleboro.)

TABLE 6.3

Utilization Statistics—Jasper Office

Name	Specialty	2014			2013			2012		
		APPTS	P-Days	DIS	APPTS	P-Days	DIS	APPTS	P-Days	DIS
Department of Primary Care										
W. G. Chan	Pediatrics	4,604	212	78	3,324	276	90	4,125	303	90
U. Unvey	Pediatrics	4,767	234	66	4,654	267	69	4,209	291	81
N. Otter	Pediatrics	4,523	206	51	4,045	224	57	4,509	205	45
P. Quester	Pediatrics	4,033	312	75	3,978	356	76	3,956	334	79
M. Polk	OB/GYN	3,651	650	140	3,612	984	202	3,487	982	215
J. Klock	OB/GYN	3,749	607	135	3,256	1,115	256	3,356	1,138	267
L. Mustard	OB/GYN	4,317	908	245	4,450	1,102	315	4,245	1,298	335
J. Washington	Internal medicine	3,745	712	156	2,867	505	101	2,456	536	146
E. Frost*	Internal medicine	4,980	700	176	3,156	646	120	2,077	495	103
L. Coolidge**	ENT	3,369	345	123	3,278	806	323	1,433	345	143
K. Kipstein	Cardiology	4,126	612	145	3,682	700	156	3,933	596	133
O. Maeer	Cardiology	4,682	698	167	4,356	512	102	4,631	878	175
	Subtotals	**50,546**	**6,196**	**1,557**	**44,658**	**7,493**	**1,867**	**42,417**	**7,401**	**1,812**
Department of Surgery										
C. Finn	General	1,587	806	165	1,601	1,206	245	700	830	203
A. Steve	Orthpedic	1,266	612	134	1,534	733	167	793	723	154
S. Lee	Orthpedic	2,156	885	231	1,935	893	287	1,689	1,104	303
L. Picture	Orthpedic	1,920	957	245	1,756	1,234	298	2,156	1,556	366
L. Goldwater	Orthpedic	2,877	1,134	278	2,645	1,376	325	2,034	1,589	387
	Subtotals	**9,806**	**4,394**	**1,053**	**9,471**	**5,442**	**1,322**	**7,372**	**5,802**	**1,413**
	Total	**60,352**	**10,590**	**2,610**	**54,129**	**12,935**	**3,189**	**49,789**	**13,203**	**3,225**

NOTES: APPTS = Appointments
P-Days = Patient days (all hospitals)
DIS = Discharges (all hospitals)
* = Hired March 1, 2012
** = Hired July 1, 2012

(This table can also be found online at ache.org/books/Middleboro.)

Department	Location	Discharges		Patient Days	
		All	HC	All	HC
Primary care	Middleboro	1,989	1,950	8,591	8,209
Surgery	Middleboro	1,378	1,323	6,885	6,192
Subtotal		**3,367**	**3,273**	**15,476**	**14,401**
Primary care	Jasper	1,557	650	6,196	1,647
Surgery	Jasper	1,053	263	4,394	1,318
Subtotal		**2,610**	**913**	**10,590**	**2,965**
Total		**5,977**	**4,186**	**26,066**	**17,366**

TABLE 6.4
Hospital Utilization Statistics by Office Location, Department, and Hospital Location (12-Month Period Ending December 31, 2014)

NOTES: All = All Hospitals
HC = Hospitals located in Hillsboro County (MCH and WH)

Physician Name	Specialty	Office	Salary ($)	Date Hired
K. Kessler	Internal medicine	Middleboro	203,000	1-Jul-13
E. Frost	Internal medicine	Jasper	206,000	1-Mar-12
L. Coolidge	ENT	Jasper	226,450	1-Jul-12

TABLE 6.5
Staff Physicians as of December 31, 2014

NOTE: Staff physicians are hired on a two-year contract

TABLE 6.6

Physician
Compensation for
2014 ($)

Name	Specialty	Draw/Salary	Benefits	Total
Chan	Pediatrics	182,450	35,760	218,210
Otter	Pediatrics	184,294	36,122	220,416
Quester	Pediatrics	185,289	36,317	221,606
Reeper	Pediatrics	182,353	35,741	218,094
Samuels	Pediatrics	193,245	37,876	231,121
St. James	Pediatrics	188,223	36,892	225,115
Unvey	Pediatrics	188,446	36,935	225,381
Dustin	OB/GYN	298,467	58,500	356,967
Gost	OB/GYN	30,348	5,948	36,296
Klock	OB/GYN	274,278	53,758	328,036
Mustard	OB/GYN	299,292	58,661	357,953
Polk	OB/GYN	288,778	56,600	345,378
Barton	Internal medicine	195,404	38,299	233,703
Douglas	Internal medicine	200,393	39,277	239,670
Frost	Internal medicine	223,445	43,795	267,240
Kessler	Internal medicine	203,272	39,841	243,113
Lesko	Internal medicine	190,704	37,378	228,082
Master	Internal medicine	195,797	38,376	234,173
Washington	Internal medicine	202,350	39,661	242,011
Kipstein	Cardiology	324,366	63,576	387,942
Maeer	Cardiology	355,378	69,654	425,032
Underwood	Cardiology	331,245	64,924	396,169
Eason	Urology	345,248	67,669	412,917
Fixer	Urology	356,340	69,843	426,183
Autumn	Gastroenterology	282,340	55,339	337,679

(continued)

Name	Specialty	Draw/Salary	Benefits	Total
Coolidge	ENT	360,300	70,619	430,919
Xerox	ENT	355,340	69,647	424,987
Weckenson	ENT	350,249	68,649	418,898
Finn	General surgery	478,330	93,753	572,083
Hersh	General surgery	354,220	69,427	423,647
Jackson	General surgery	372,454	73,001	445,455
Never	General surgery	451,665	88,526	540,191
O'Connell	General surgery	424,200	83,143	507,343
Putter	General surgery	475,334	93,165	568,499
Goldwater	Orthopedic surgery	405,778	79,532	485,310
Lee	Orthopedic surgery	447,560	87,722	535,282
Picture	Orthopedic surgery	451,800	88,553	540,353
Qestrom	Orthopedic surgery	406,002	79,576	485,578
Stanley	Orthopedic surgery	407,219	79,815	487,034
Steve	Orthopedic surgery	525,330	102,965	628,295
	Total	12,167,526	2,384,835	14,552,361

TABLE 6.6
Physician Compensation for 2014 ($) (continued)

NOTE: Does not include compensation for administrative and management duties and responsibilities

TABLE 6.7

Statement of Revenue and Expenses for Calendar Years Ending December 31 ($)

	2014	2013	2012
Revenue			
Patient services revenue	46,732,370	41,961,328	39,295,973
Allowance	8,206,111	7,658,241	5,720,365
Bad debt	760,040	519,476	498,207
Net patient services revenue	37,766,219	33,783,611	33,077,401
Other operating revenue	8,070	3,026	7,456
Total operating revenue	**37,774,289**	**33,786,637**	**33,084,857**
Expenses			
Physician compensation	14,552,361	14,088,994	13,455,329
Other professional services	15,681,186	13,425,397	13,327,203
General services	3,548,975	2,243,109	2,125,242
Fiscal services	1,739,871	1,610,224	1,428,305
Interest	185,523	179,058	174,894
Depreciation	1,841,231	1,997,170	2,361,678
Total operating expenses	**37,549,147**	**33,543,952**	**32,872,651**
Pretax income (loss)	225,142	242,685	212,206
Taxes	85,554	92,220	80,638
Profit (loss)	**139,588**	**150,465**	**131,568**

(This table can also be found online at ache.org/books/Middleboro.)

	2014	2013	2012
Assets			
Current assets			
Cash and marketable securities	3,563,292	2,867,340	3,763,193
Accounts receivable—gross	8,929,737	7,423,188	7,334,868
Allowances for uncollectables	(927,353)	(689,303)	(612,039)
Accounts receivable—net	8,002,384	6,733,885	6,722,829
Due from third-party payers	556,247	634,929	1,012,745
Inventory	739,864	443,988	515,200
Prepaid expenses	254,352	797,665	342,389
Total current assets	**13,116,139**	**11,477,807**	**12,356,356**
Noncurrent assets			
Property, plant, and equipment—gross	47,159,223	47,112,343	45,182,334
Less accumulated depreciation	(19,084,473)	(17,243,242)	(15,246,072)
Property, plant, and equipment—net	28,074,750	29,869,101	29,936,262
Other investments	1,917,234	2,120,940	2,087,230
Total assets	**43,108,123**	**43,467,848**	**44,379,848**

TABLE 6.8
Balance Sheet as
of December 31 ($)

(continued)

TABLE 6.8
Balance Sheet as
of December 31 ($)
(continued)

	2014	2013	2012
Liabilities			
Current liabilities			
Accounts payable	2,143,485	1,882,494	1,701,905
Accrued salaries and wages	837,240	801,282	735,240
Accrued interest	180,238	200,345	210,876
Other accrued expenses	137,450	154,203	150,239
Accrued vacation days	92,867	90,124	84,236
Due to third-party vendors	198,335	100,000	81,564
Long-term debt due within one year	952,189	874,230	912,572
Total current liabilities	**4,541,804**	**4,102,678**	**3,876,632**
Long-term debt	5,229,449	6,167,888	7,456,399
Total liabilities	**9,771,253**	**10,270,566**	**11,333,031**
Net assets	33,336,870	33,197,282	33,046,817
Total liabilities and net assets	**43,108,123**	**43,467,848**	**44,379,848**

(This table can also be found online at ache.org/books/Middleboro.)

Month	Total Cases	Weekdays	Type of Cases	
			ENT	Ortho and Other
January	81	11	47	34
February	149	19	89	60
March	167	21	94	73
April	199	22	110	89
May	203	21	121	82
June	204	21	120	84
July	222	22	133	89
August	221	21	128	93
September	216	21	113	103
October	261	23	147	114
November	268	17	103	165
December	257	17	109	148
Total	2,448	236	1,314	1,134

TABLE 6.9

Operational Statistics for Ambulatory Surgery in Jasper for the 12 Months Ending December 31, 2014

NOTE: During this period, Ambulatory Surgery used two operating suites. One was devoted to ENT and the other to orthopedics and other procedures. The unit began serving patients on January 16, 2014.

Weekdays = Number of operational days in the month, excludes holidays

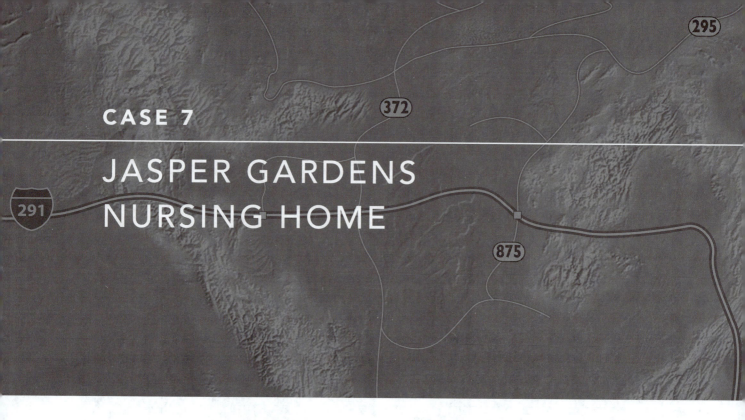

CASE 7

JASPER GARDENS NURSING HOME

Jasper Gardens is a for-profit nursing home located on east side of Jasper, about five miles from the city center. The facility is a one-story modern building with ample parking and significant room for expansion. It is located near Medical Associates on 65 acres of land adjacent to the newly approved highway, approximately one mile from the planned Jasper–East exit. Jasper Gardens is licensed to operate 110 beds. It currently operates and staffs 106 beds in both private and semi-private rooms,

JEFFERSON PARTNERS, LLC

Jasper Gardens is owned and operated by Jefferson Partners, LLC. This corporation owns and operates nursing homes, assisted living facilities, retirement living communities, and adult day care centers in the greater Capital City area and statewide. Jefferson Partners is a private equity partnership of investors. None of the investors is involved in the day-to-day management of the corporation. The partners have quarterly board meetings, and their executive committee meets monthly with the professional senior management team to review operations and issues. Jefferson Partners acquired the Jasper Gardens property in 1995 and has continuously invested in the property.

Jefferson Partners has two operating divisions: property and management. The management division provides centralized administrative services, such as payroll, legal services, financial management, and group purchasing for its facilities, and it also charges a management fee for its services.

The property division owns the buildings and land, and it leases these properties to wholly owned subsidiary corporations that manage the individual operations. As such, Jasper Gardens leases its current building and land.

The senior management team of Jefferson Partners includes Ralph Jefferson, president and CEO, and Mary Charles, RN, vice president of operations. David Fellows is the director of corporate development and acquisitions. Martha Wyman is the chief financial officer. The senior management team/central office approves the annual budget for each facility. Charles meets monthly with facility administrators to monitor operations and to address problems and issues. Jefferson Partners maintains professional offices and a small, central staff in Capital City.

HISTORY

The Jasper Gardens Nursing Home traces its history back to 1960, when it was founded by Mary and John Decker. The initial facility was a former resort that accommodated 45 residents in semiprivate rooms. During the 1970s this facility was modified to accommodate 70 residents and was licensed under the Medicaid and Medicare programs. In 1980, the Deckers sold the facility to the Armstrong family, who then built four new wings of patient rooms, each with 12 semiprivate rooms. On each occasion, the state awarded a Certificate of Need (CON). This construction project (1981 to 1983) used the original structure for administrative offices and common areas.

Between 1990 and 1995, the facility was modified into its current configuration with five wings and a central building for administrative patient care. In this modification, the original resort house structure was demolished and totally replaced. The original four wings were updated and modified. Jefferson Partners acquired the facility in 1995. Today the structure is modern and tastefully decorated to emphasize the residential nature of a contemporary nursing home.

Until 1992 the state CON law regulated any expansion in nursing homes that cost more than $500,000. Today the threshold for nursing homes is the same as for acute care facilities. In 1992 the state also ceased allowing any nursing home to expand its bed capacity 5 percent each year without a CON, regardless of cost. It should be noted that capital costs are capped and used to determine state Medicaid rates for nursing homes; they constitute less than 5 percent to a rate calculation. Currently, the state has placed a moratorium on CON applications for skilled nursing facility and intermediate care facility beds pending changes in the state CON law. However, the governor has granted permission that the number of beds in a nursing home may increase if the total number of nursing home beds within a county remains unchanged.

When Jasper Gardens was originally founded, the surrounding area was relatively rural. Today it is becoming more suburban, and a number of housing developments have been built nearby. A shopping center is located approximately a quarter-mile away. The area is expected to grow and develop significantly with the opening of the new interstate road between Jasper and Capital City.

The facility introduced Resident Community Councils in 2007, which give residents opportunities to meet with the staff to express their wishes and preferences. Jasper Gardens has been recognized as a regional leader in empowering residents and creating a homelike atmosphere. Its promotion materials stress this and cite many examples:

> The residents have choices with respect to how they want to live. We promise to listen and strive to accommodate resident choices so that we can fulfill their wishes for daily living. A "fine dining" program is available to a different group of residents daily. We create a restaurant-like atmosphere here with fine china, silverware, and food and personal service. Residents go to local restaurants regularly in groups, by themselves, or bring food back to their rooms for private dining. Bathing or showering times are honored by request for time, day, and frequency. Staff members have consistent assignments of residents for continuity of care and familiarity of daily routines for residents. The facility makes available its facilities and space to the community for meetings and social functions.

For the past four years, Jasper Gardens has been a semifinalist in the statewide competition for the Quality-of-Life Award granted by the governor to the nursing home best able to demonstrate its commitment to resident independence and to giving patients choices regarding their care and services.

PATIENT SERVICES

Jasper Gardens is licensed by the state to operate 110 nursing home beds. It accepts all forms of payment. It is 100 percent Medicare- and Medicaid-certified and fully approved to provide skilled nursing and rehabilitation services covered by Medicare. Medicaid covers most patients. Physical therapy (PT), occupational therapy (OT), recreation therapy, and speech therapy (ST) services are available onsite. These rehabilitation services are also available to area citizens as outpatients. These outpatients use either Medicare Part B or commercial insurance to cover associated charges.

Jasper Gardens classifies its patients and residents and many of its services using "intermediate care" and "skilled care." The term *resident* implies an individual with an average length of stay (ALOS) of more than three months, whereas the term *patient* means an individual with an ALOS of fewer than 100 days. Intermediate care services emphasize long-term residual services. In 2014, the ALOS for intermediate care patients is 2.8 years and has been increasing. The average age of current residents is 87 and has slowly been increasing. Some residents in this category have the ability to pay for care when they are initially admitted. Many, however, after spending down their available personal resources, have their care financed by Medicaid. The average spend-down period for the residents of Jasper Gardens, over the past five years, has dropped from 16 months to 13 months. A few patients in this category are covered by private nursing home insurance or insurance provided by the US Department of Veterans Affairs.

Skilled care patients are in the nursing home for post-hospital rehabilitation. Patients older than 65 years of age rely on Medicare as their primary insurance. These patients make use of PT, OT, and ST services. Those not eligible for Medicare typically rely on a private health insurance plan to cover these services. In 2014 the ALOS for Medicare patients was 36.2 days; it has been decreasing over the past five years. However, 40 percent of Medicare patients stay beyond 60 days. For patients covered by private or commercial health insurance, the ALOS in 2014 was 24.3 days.

Registered nurses (RNs), licensed practical nurses (LPNs), licensed nursing assistants (LNAs), and medication nursing assistants (MNAs) provide nursing services. A part-time registered dietitian supervises all food services. Social work services are provided during the admissions process and are available on an in-patient basis. Pharmacy services are provided on contract by DRUGCO, Inc.

The medical director is James A. Child, DO. He is board certified in family practice and gerontology, and he operates a practice in Jasper with Drs. Freda Evans and David Dodger. Drs. Evans and Dodger provide backup on-call services at Jasper Gardens as needed. All three are active medical staff members at Webster Hospital and have consulting medical staff privileges at Osteopathic Medical Center in Capital City. Dr. Child devotes approximately one day per week to his patients in Jasper Gardens.

The facility is physically divided into five adjacent wings. Four of the five wings have nine semiprivate rooms and two private rooms. The facility has eight private rooms in total. These four wings were part of the original 1980 construction and have been modified over the years to accommodate larger lounges and patient common areas. The fifth wing, added in 1995, has 13 semiprivate rooms and houses the rehabilitation services department. Each wing also has a nursing station, a shower room, and a small library. Wireless Internet is available throughout the entire facility. The beauty salon and barbershop are located in the central commons area. Most patients enter Jasper Gardens following discharge from an area hospital. Primary referral sources include the hospitals located in Middleboro and Capital City.

ORGANIZATION

Jasper Gardens is organized using a flat management structure. The senior management team reports to the administrator who in turn reports to Mary Charles, the vice president of operations for Jefferson Partners LLC (located in Capital City). The senior management team meets weekly to review the budget reports furnished by Jefferson Partners. Each of the senior managers supervises and directs multiple departments and staff.

Jayne Winters, NHA, is the licensed administrator of Jasper Gardens. She is a graduate of an eastern university and holds an undergraduate degree in health services management. On her graduation in 2006, she completed her administrator-in-training program at a Jefferson Partners facility in Capital City. Upon completion of this program, she earned her state license and was appointed as assistant administrator at Jefferson Partners' largest nursing home, an assisted living and congregate living (apartment) facility in Capital City. She was appointed administrator of Jasper Gardens in 2010. Winters is active in the statewide association of long-term care administrators and lives in Jasper. Winters also manages all aspects of personnel and human resources administration. For example, her office releases all advertisements for employment and screens all applicants. Wage and salary rates are set during the annual budgeting process, with changes requiring the approval of Jefferson Partners. Winters and her administrative assistant, Carol Hyde, administer all employment (including employment background checks) and benefit policies.

Over the past 18 months, employees have filed formal grievances related to "unfair interpretations" involving annual and sick leave policies, merit pay adjustments, and rates paid to part-time workers who work on national holidays. During this same period, three employees were discharged for failure to perform stated duties. It should be noted that one of Winters's first actions as administrator was the dismissal of three employees for nepotism. This action is still remembered by many of the staff, who felt the dismissals were not necessary, especially because these employees were hired before a formal policy on nepotism was instituted. Recently two other employees were discharged for poor attendance and work performance. Winters is also responsible for all advertising and promotional programs designed to call attention to the facility.

When interviewed, Winters indicated that Medicaid pricing has continued to force Jasper Gardens to carefully reconsider all staffing levels and in some instances to reduce staffing. She indicated that any nursing home—and especially Jasper Gardens—works within slim annual financial margins and that small staffing increases could easily evaporate its modest profitability. She also indicated that her employment contract does include certain incentives and penalties related to quality of care and financial performance.

When asked to identify and discuss significant issues, she noted that for the past two years Jasper Gardens has received a deficiency-free survey from the state Department of Health–Level B. This, she explained, is a significant improvement over the conditions that existed when she was hired. Prior to 2010, the state survey team awarded Jasper Gardens scores that indicated widespread potential for more than minimal harm to patients (Levels E and F). Winters stated that the positive surveys over the past three years were the result of a solid and dedicated team effort and changes in some job responsibilities. She also indicated that, over her four-year career at Jasper Gardens, patient acuity and levels of need have increased: "The intensity of needed care has increased significantly. More and more of our older residents are exhibiting behavioral problems. Even though our staffing has remained about the same, our residents seem to need more and more care."

Three years ago, Jasper Gardens' workers' compensation rates doubled based on its history of worker injuries. The most common injury has been back strains and pulls associated with assisting and lifting residents from their beds. During 2014, because of new policies and the arrival of new equipment to help staff assist residents, no staff member reported back injuries.

No union has ever represented the hourly staff at Jasper Gardens. Unofficially, Winters did indicate that she and her management team have heard rumors that a local union in Capital City will be sending cards to the hourly staff to determine whether the staff wants the union to represent their interests. A union formally approached the staff four years ago. If a sufficient number of cards are returned to the union, it will petition the state labor board for permission to hold an election and form a bargaining unit.

A number of residents use electric wheelchairs and carts for transportation around the nursing home and use them to frequent the small park on the grounds of the facility. In two instances over the past 18 months, "crashes" inside the facility have injured three residents. As the area has developed with wider roads and sidewalks, a small number of residents also have begun to use their personal mobility carts to go to the local shopping center. To leave the building and grounds of Jasper Gardens, a resident must secure permission from the supervising nurse and take a wireless phone furnished by the nursing home. Legal counsel is reviewing this practice to ensure that it is in keeping with current laws and regulations. Two different families have requested that the residents be restricted to using the carts only on the property of the nursing home. Current policies do not allow for these restrictions unless they are based on appropriate legal (e.g., power of attorney) or medical orders. Medicare purchases these carts for any mobility-impaired individual who is 65 years old or older. Recently an ambulatory resident, who had walked to a local shopping center, became disoriented and had to be brought back to Jasper Gardens by the police. This is the fifth such instance within the past six months.

When interviewed, Winters said:

I am very pleased with the progress we have made here over the past four years. The facility looks good, the staff is dedicated, and the owners are comfortable with our [profit] margins. We have been challenged to get our personnel system in better shape and have been responsive to needs of our workers. I sincerely hope that we do not unionize, although we fully support our employees' rights in this area. I know that Jefferson Partners is going to want us to continue to develop this facility. Especially with the new interstate road, which will significantly cut down on the travel time between Jasper and Capital City, we may have the potential for open senior living apartments and an assisted-living facility here on our current campus. We have the space and a great deal of the infrastructure to move in this direction.

When asked about the management reports she relies on, Winters said that her "dashboard report" is critical to her ability to stay abreast of the management issues in the facility. This weekly report includes the following information for the latest week, month, quarter, and year to date:

◆ Revenue and expense budget performance

◆ Payroll information: budgeted versus actual hours, dollars, and overtime

◆ Patient census by payer

◆ Admissions and discharges

◆ Therapy revenue, expenses, and hours

◆ Employee health insurance claims submitted

◆ Primary quality indicators:

— Facility-acquired pressure ulcers

— Falls

— Injuries

— Weight loss

— Reportable events

— Acute discharges

Michele Regan, RN, is director of nursing and patient services at Jasper Gardens. She holds an undergraduate degree in nursing and master's degree in geriatric nursing. She has more than 20 years of professional experience in long-term care nursing. She joined the nursing staff at Jasper Gardens as the day-shift charge nurse in 2004. She was appointed to her current position in 2009. She supervises the day (7:00 a.m.–3:00 p.m.), evening (3:00 p.m.–11:00 p.m.), and night (11:00 p.m.–7:00 a.m.) nursing supervisors. There are two day-shift charge nurses. Each is responsible for approximately half of the patients. Aside from supervising all nursing services, Regan also supervises the ancillary services unit (i.e., PT, OT, ST, and respiratory therapy) and the recreation unit, and she coordinates all pharmaceutical services. When interviewed she discussed staffing and management issues. She indicated that (surprisingly) Jasper Gardens rarely has experienced any problem hiring qualified RNs and LPNs. She indicated that Jasper Gardens experiences the expected turnover in its LNA workforce and that she would like to hire more MNAs when LNA openings occur. She also indicated that staff scheduling was always an issue: "We seem to be in a catch-22. Recently we have begun to hire more part-time staff. But scheduling them and relying on them to work a few extra hours to help us cover a shift here and there has been difficult and disappointing. In the past we hired some floating full-time staff to cover as needed, but we moved to part-time staff to save money. This move seems to have made staffing much more difficult. It appears that the critical complaint of our part-time staff is that they do not have sick leave, something very important to them when they have sick children."

Regan did speak positively about the certified therapeutic recreation specialists who now staff the recreation department. Jasper Gardens began hiring certified specialists in this department four years ago, and it has "led to our recreation services department being one of the best in the state."

Working with the medical director, Dr. Child, Regan is also responsible for the formulary, ensuring that adequate pharmacy stock is maintained and that appropriate inventory safeguards are effective. She is responsible for the ordering and inventory of all medical supplies. Medical supplies are purchased using contracts negotiated and administered by Jefferson Partners.

When asked what changes she would like to see, she stated, "Our current policy concerning residents being hospitalized and then returning may need to be reconsidered." She stated, "Our current policy is that we will not keep a bed open for a resident who is admitted to a hospital unless they pay for it during their hospitalization or absence. If the bed is not paid for, we will refill it after 24 hours. We also have a 10-day limit on how long any bed may be unoccupied even if the per diem charges are being paid." She continued, "This can really cause problems for our residents, but we need to keep our beds full. The situation is just not good for our residents, even though it might be a required business practice. We really try to accommodate our residents, but frequently we can't." She also indicated that a plan to dedicate one wing to patients with Alzheimer's disease and dementia, an idea recently discussed with the owners, might be needed and that such a wing would expand the range of patient care services offered.

Margaret Hemp is the director of admissions and social services. She has an undergraduate degree and a master's degree in social work and more than 15 years of professional experience. Prior to her appointment as director of admissions in 1999, she held a similar position at another nursing home in Capital City. She meets with all prospective residents and their families. She also helps potential and current residents qualify for Medicaid. Periodically she leads the team that reviews the medical and social needs of all residents, and she files reports as needed. Each resident maintains a modest cash account to support certain purchases (e.g., beauty shop). Hemp manages this system in keeping with federal and state regulations. Aside from working with the discharge teams at the hospitals located in Middleboro and Capital City, she also has regular contact with the Hillsboro County Home Health Agency and the home health agencies located in Capital City. When interviewed, she stated:

Overall, Jasper Gardens is not unique. We have a dedicated staff. Our resident population is getting older, and recent Medicare admissions have required significantly more therapy and services than in the past. Changing federal and state regulations covering Medicaid eligibility make aspects of my job demanding. I spend a great deal of time completing the minimum data set on residents to be admitted, and I spend time with our nursing supervisors filing reports on our current residents.

We really do reflect the community we serve. Our residents, for the most part, come from right around here, although the new interstate should bring us even more Capital City residents. We are fortunate that a significant number of our residents have family and friends in the area who still visit them. We seem to have more visitors than other homes that I am aware of. I enjoy working here.

Ralph Doyle is the director of plant operations. He is responsible for all aspects of the physical facility, including maintenance, laundry, and housekeeping services. His staff also runs the van that takes residents to appointments and on shopping trips. He retired from the military in 2004 and has served in this role at Jasper Gardens since 2006. Prior to his current employment, he was the associate director of facilities at another nursing home in Capital City. Under Doyle's leadership, Jasper Gardens has received no negative reports or citations regarding any aspect of facility, including fire safety inspections. In 2011, Jasper Gardens installed new onsite generators. Jasper Gardens has the ability to function "off the electric grid" for a maximum of 12 days. This addition completed a plan to make this home energy independent to ensure the safety of all residents.

When interviewed he stated:

Well, those electric carts—some call them scooters—really cause us problems. Most can't be stored inside the facility because of existing regulations covering their recharging. We have had to develop a space in another building for their storage, and we bring them in and out as the residents want them. Maybe they should be banned, especially inside the facility, as they can frequently mark or damage our floors and walls. Sometimes I feel that we are running a valet service for these carts. Overall, this is a solid facility. It is clean and relatively modern and well lighted. I am proud of how our staff has made this older facility look good. Now that we are energy independent, I sleep better at night. We also have a staff that understands our need to periodically have fire and emergency drills. This has helped a great deal. One of my many duties, however, is security. While all staff members wear badges and are instructed to question any visitors they do not know, it frequently comes down to my staff being called. I question whether we can and should remain as open as we are. Residents can potentially leave anytime they want, and outsiders can enter multiple doors from 7:00 a.m. to 8:00 p.m. before the building is "locked" for night. This may be an issue that needs attention.

It should be noted that, based on Doyle's recommendation, all residents who want to use motorized wheelchairs and carts must complete driving lessons done by a trained instructor and earn a scooter license from Jasper Gardens.

Bonnie Keana is the senior administrative assistant and bookkeeper. She is responsible for preparing the payroll and supervising the posting of the financial journal and the general ledger. Based on information she prepares, Jefferson Partners provides budget status reports every week and interim financial statements monthly. Keana is also in charge of local purchasing, and she supervises the reception staff.

MANAGEMENT OPERATIONS

Every Tuesday morning, Winters, Regan, and Hemp meet to review the status of all patients. Data include quality measures used by the Medicare Quality Improvement Organization and Centers for Medicare & Medicaid Services (CMS) as well as other data reported to Jefferson Partners. Once a month this committee includes others (including the medical director) as needed from its Continuous Quality Improvement Committee and reviews all data to determine which patients and CMS items need attention, why, and the treatment and prevention approaches being used.

Every Friday morning, Winters, Regan, and Hemp plus Doyle and Keana meet as the management team and review the most recent dashboard report, budget status report, and other issues needing management's attention.

CURRENT ISSUES

PERSONNEL AND UNION ACTIVITY

When interviewed, Winters and Regan both indicated that access to qualified professional staff was not a major problem. They stated, "We have been able to hire highly qualified professionals who have generally stayed with us for significant periods of time." Over the years, however, some wages have not kept pace with the regional market. This trend has been directly traceable to Medicaid rates paid by the state. Over the past ten years, state Medicaid rates have fallen from being the tenth highest in the United States to the eighth lowest.

Four years ago, the hourly employees were mailed cards and met regularly with union organizers from Capital City. This effort did not yield a sufficient number of staff to petition to form a bargaining unit. Two years ago, as part of study done by an external consultant, employees expressed three primary job concerns. They were concerned that wages were below market norms, that benefits were administered unfairly, and that job expectations were unclear. After this study, Jefferson Partners did authorize some wage changes and committed to follow a standardized system of benefits for all employees. This system is described in a new and expanded employee manual, which has not yet been published. The study also instructed the administrator to review and update all job descriptions and to enhance the system of annual evaluation. Merit pay was introduced in 2013 but has met with mixed reviews and results. Four years ago, the personnel system was ad hoc and poorly defined. It still exhibits a number of shortcomings. For example, a number of employees remain confused about their eligibility for certain benefits and how to use benefits.

REHABILITATION SERVICES UTILIZATION

Rehabilitation services (i.e., PT, OT, ST, and respiratory therapy) are available for nursing home residents as well as members of the community. Most pay for these services using Medicare Part B or private insurance. Outpatient utilization continues to be almost nonexistent. Currently, individuals in need of ambulatory rehabilitation services typically travel to either Capital City or Middleboro. Jefferson Partners has asked Jasper Gardens for a plan to address this potential market as part of the upcoming review of the draft budget for 2016.

Jasper Gardens estimates that for 2015, service demands (in relative value units, or RVUs) will be 5,000 units in PT, 7,500 units in OT, and 700 units in ST. Space exists to address the needs of more patients. Note that workers' compensation provides an annual limit of up to 24 PT and/or OT visit per year per injury. Jasper Gardens' 2015 staffing devoted to providing patient services (in FTEs) for this department will be

- ◆   1.0 PT,

- ◆   0.3 physical therapy assistant,

- ◆   1.0 OT,

- ◆   0.7 certified occupational therapy assistant, and

- ◆   0.3 ST.

Note that the supervisor of this department splits her time between administration and providing PT services. Jefferson Partners has a target that 90 percent of available time in a rehab unit be devoted to patient care.

Increasingly, institutional profitability is based on the success of the SNF unit and outpatient rehabilitation services. Medicaid rates covering the ICF make it difficult to achieve institutional profitability.

ADMISSION POLICIES

Beginning in 2014, Jefferson Partners has required that all nursing home patient and resident applicants submit to a background check as a condition associated with admission. Jefferson Partners has indicated that no potential patient or resident with a felony conviction as a sexual predator or offender will be admitted. This policy is explained to all potential patients and residents. Jasper Gardens has implemented this policy at all of its facilities. It should be noted that this policy is under legal review at two of Jefferson Partners' other nursing homes.

SPECIAL PROGRAMS AND NEW INITIATIVES

Hospice Care with Capital City VNA

Capital City VNA and Hospice has proposed that a collaborative Medicare-certified inpatient hospice be established at Jasper Gardens. This hospice would serve the greater Jasper community and provide access to these services to the Medicare-eligible population. Currently, Jasper residents requesting the use of Medicare-certified hospice services must seek care in Capital City. Capital City VNA and Hospice would enter into a contractual relationship with Jasper Gardens for private rooms to be used for inpatient hospice care. The medical director of the hospice would supervise and direct the cases, and nurses from the hospice would be assigned to provide 24-hour care, with support and extra coverage provided by the staff of the nursing home as needed.

Jasper Gardens is able to do this under existing Medicare regulations involving its SNF. It could provide all staffing and direct patient services in this new unit. It could provide a dedicated wing, area, or building with private rooms for the patients, meals, general nursing supervision, and general services (such as housekeeping). Capital City VNA (potentially the Medicare-certified hospice) would pay Jasper Gardens (as a subcontractor) a price per patient day to be negotiated. Direct service costs would be approximately $75 per day for the requested services. Jasper Gardens' pharmacy service would provide needed drugs and other durable medical equipment at cost that would be directly reimbursed to the pharmacy by Capital City VNA and Hospice. The initial estimate is that Jasper Gardens could add a new dedicated wing of four to eight private rooms at approximately $150,000 per private room (minimum of four).

Assisted Living Facility and Retirement Housing

Jefferson Partners has included in its strategic plan the development of many more services on the campus of Jasper Gardens. The company is interested in an assisted living facility, congregate living facility (senior apartments), and retirement housing adjacent to Jasper Gardens. The idea is to use the land currently owned by Jefferson Partners, a location that should be very attractive given the new interstate highway to be opened. This plan would designate the nursing home administrator as the campus CEO. The CEO would be responsible for the facilities on the campus. Staffing would be adjusted as needed so that Jasper Gardens' employees would provide staffing for the new facilities.

Jefferson Partners is currently determining cost estimates for these types of facilities and hopes to have a conceptual plan ready for its architects within six months. It estimates that the assisted living facility would cost approximately $300 per square foot and that apartments and housing would cost around $200 per square foot. The Jasper Planning Board has indicated that current zoning would make this type of adult senior community a "natural addition" to the nursing home campus. The added taxes also would help the town defray the costs of infrastructure development (i.e., roads, water, and sewer) that it embarked on three years ago. Jefferson Partners has identified two significant questions to be resolved—what is the best size, and what are the associated costs of this plan? The company has indicated that it will complete the market and financial feasibility study for this project in 2015. Some studies suggest that the average length of rental in an assisted living facility is 5.4 years, with a standard deviation of 2.3 years. National studies suggest that these types of facilities are attractive to specific segments of the population.

Information System Developments

Jefferson Partners has recently signed a contract with Nursing Home Systems, Inc., to install—companywide—an electronic health record system. Training should begin in nine months, and the system should be fully installed and implemented by December 2015. The system will be a comprehensive medical record with order entry for supplies, tests, and all medically related activities. Jefferson Partners estimates that this system will cost approximately $2,000 per bed to install.

Unrelated to the development of the electronic health record system is the recent request from Osteopathic Medical Center (OMC) in Capital City to partner in a tele-health system. Under this system a nursing home patient at Jasper Gardens could be evaluated and cared for by an attending physician at OMC. The system should preclude the physical transfer of some nursing home patients to OMC for diagnosis and treatment. Note that if a patient is medically transferred to a hospital, the nursing home can refill the empty bed after 24 hours. No cost estimate for this system is available.

Potential Need and Demand for Alzheimer's and Dementia Wing

Jefferson Partners has requested that the staff assess the need and demand for a wing dedicated to serving patients with Alzheimer's disease or dementia. It has asked the staff to examine options and to indicate characteristics of this unit (e.g., secured versus unsecured) as well as unique staffing and care needs. Jefferson Partners has requested that this analysis be provided before any decision is made concerning additional construction on the site.

The following tables provide more information about Jasper Gardens' patients, residents, financial status, staffing, and quality measures.

	2014	2013	2012	2011	2010	2009	2008
Type of Primary Insurance							
Skilled care							
Medicare	24	26	24	30	22	26	25
Commercial	1	2	3	1	2	1	1
Intermediate care							
Medicaid	60	63	60	63	63	56	60
Veterans Affairs	1	2	2	1	1	3	2
Private insurance	1	0	0	1	1	1	0
Self-pay	12	8	7	5	10	12	9
Total number of beds	106	106	106	106	106	106	106
Total filled beds	99	101	96	101	99	99	97
Facility occupancy	93.4%	95.3%	90.6%	95.3%	93.4%	93.4%	91.5%

TABLE 7.1
Patient Census by Type of Insurance as of December 31

Number	Age	Gender	Months	Comm	Ins	Ref	S or I
1	99	2	81.0	9	2	4	I
2	99	2	88.0	5	2	2	I
3	98	2	32.0	9	2	3	I
4	97	2	75.0	9	2	2	I
5	96	1	41.0	1	2	3	I
6	96	2	30.0	3	2	4	I
7	94	2	21.0	1	2	2	I
8	94	2	27.0	3	2	2	I
9	93	2	76.0	5	2	1	I
10	93	2	17.0	3	2	4	I
11	93	2	34.0	2	2	5	I
12	93	1	25.0	3	2	2	I
13	92	2	31.0	1	2	3	I

TABLE 7.2
Resident Information as of December 31, 2014

(continued)

TABLE 7.2
Resident Information as of December 31, 2014 (continued)

Number	Age	Gender	Months	Comm	Ins	Ref	S or I
14	92	2	20.0	3	2	5	I
15	92	2	73.0	9	2	1	I
16	91	2	84.0	5	2	1	I
17	90	2	1.0	5	1	4	S
18	90	2	72.0	5	2	2	I
19	90	2	56.0	5	2	2	I
20	90	2	24.0	5	2	1	I
21	90	2	30.0	9	2	3	I
22	90	1	23.0	1	2	6	I
23	90	2	19.0	3	2	2	I
24	90	2	19.0	3	2	6	I
25	90	2	39.0	3	2	1	I
26	90	1	48.0	3	2	1	I
27	89	1	0.8	5	1	6	S
28	89	2	23.0	9	2	4	I
29	89	2	24.0	3	2	2	I
30	89	1	38.0	3	2	1	I
31	89	2	22.0	3	2	6	I
32	89	1	60.0	3	2	1	I
33	89	2	4.0	2	2	5	I
34	89	2	30.0	9	2	3	I
35	88	2	2.0	3	1	1	S
36	88	2	1.0	5	1	2	S
37	88	2	38.0	3	2	2	I
38	88	1	30.0	3	2	2	I
39	88	2	5.0	3	2	5	I
40	88	2	24.0	9	2	6	I
41	88	2	26.0	9	2	5	I

(continued)

Number	Age	Gender	Months	Comm	Ins	Ref	S or I
42	88	1	35.0	3	2	1	I
43	87	2	30.0	5	2	1	I
44	87	2	21.0	9	2	6	I
45	87	2	30.0	3	2	2	I
46	87	2	8.0	10	2	6	I
47	87	2	9.0	1	2	5	I
48	86	2	30.0	3	2	3	I
49	86	2	35.0	3	2	1	I
50	86	1	19.0	3	2	6	I
51	86	2	26.0	3	2	3	I
52	85	2	2.0	3	1	2	S
53	85	1	23.0	3	2	3	I
54	85	2	33.0	2	2	6	I
55	85	1	7.0	4	6	6	I
56	84	1	20.0	6	2	5	I
57	84	2	37.0	3	2	1	I
58	84	1	32.0	3	2	5	I
59	84	2	31.0	3	2	1	I
60	83	1	8.0	3	2	5	I
61	83	1	13.0	3	2	5	I
62	83	2	18.0	5	2	6	I
63	83	2	16.0	1	2	3	I
64	82	1	0.4	2	1	2	S
65	82	2	0.8	9	1	2	S
66	82	2	12.0	9	2	4	I
67	80	2	0.9	5	1	1	S
68	80	2	0.2	5	1	4	S
69	80	1	1.5	3	1	1	S

TABLE 7.2
Resident Information as of December 31, 2014 (continued)

(continued)

TABLE 7.2
Resident
Information as
of December 31,
2014
(continued)

Number	Age	Gender	Months	Comm	Ins	Ref	S or I
70	80	1	0.5	5	1	6	S
71	78	2	0.3	1	1	5	S
72	78	1	1.0	3	1	2	S
73	77	2	0.2	3	1	1	S
74	73	2	2.0	3	1	1	S
75	71	2	0.8	3	1	4	S
76	71	2	11.0	3	6	1	I
77	70	2	0.9	5	1	4	S
78	70	2	0.5	3	1	4	S
79	69	2	1.0	3	1	1	S
80	68	2	0.5	3	1	2	S
81	68	2	2.0	3	1	3	S
82	68	2	8.0	3	6	2	I
83	67	1	0.5	3	1	2	S
84	66	1	9.0	3	6	5	I
85	66	2	2.3	3	1	6	S
86	65	2	0.5	3	1	4	S
87	63	1	2.5	3	5	2	I
88	63	1	2.0	3	6	2	I
89	62	2	3.0	3	4	1	S
90	61	2	9.0	3	6	5	I
91	60	1	7.0	3	6	3	I
92	59	1	0.5	1	3	2	I
93	59	2	3.0	3	6	1	I
94	59	2	10.0	1	6	1	I
95	58	2	0.5	3	2	2	I
96	58	1	7.0	3	6	1	I
97	57	2	1.5	9	2	3	I

(continued)

TABLE 7.2
Resident
Information as
of December 31,
2014
(continued)

Number	Age	Gender	Months	Comm	Ins	Ref	S or I
98	56	2	10.0	3	6	2	I
99	28	2	12.0	2	6	1	I

NOTES:

Number = Patient ID number

Age = As of December 31

Gender: 1 = Male; 2 = Female

Months = Months in residence

Comm = Community of origin:

  1 Middleboro

  2 Mifflenville

  3 Jasper

  4 Harris City

  5 Statesville

  6 Carterville

  7 Boalsburg

  8 Minortown

  9 Capital City

 10 Other

Ins = Insurance

  1 Medicare

  2 Medicaid

  3 Veterans Affairs

  4 Commercial

  5 Other private

  6 Self-pay

Ref = Referral

  1 Middleboro Community Hospital

  2 Webster Hospital

  3 Osteopathic Medical Center

  4 Other Capital City hospital

  5 From home

  6 Other

S = Skilled care

I = Intermediate care

TABLE 7.3
FTE Staffing as of
December 31

		2014	2013
Administration	Administrator	1.0	1.0
	Payroll supervisor*	1.0	1.0
	Receptionist*	1.0	0.8
Maintenance	Supervisor	1.0	1.0
	Staff*	0.5	0.6
Housekeeping	Supervisor	1.0	1.0
	Staff*	5.3	5.5
	Laundry assistants*	2.6	2.8

(continued)

TABLE 7.3
FTE Staffing as
of December 31
(continued)

		2014	2013
Dietary	Supervisor	0.4	1.0
	Dietician, director	0.5	0.5
	Cooks*	2.9	2.9
	Assistants*	6.7	6.5
Nursing	Director	1.0	1.0
	MDS coordinator	1.0	1.0
	Staff development coordinator	1.0	1.0
	RN supervisor	2.6	2.6
	RN charge*	6.2	6.3
	LPN charge*	9.3	9.2
	Certified nursing assistants*	37.8	38.2
	Medical technologists*	1.3	1.3
	Medical records*	0.8	0.8
Recreation	Supervisor	1.0	1.0
	Staff*	2.0	2.2
Social services	Supervisor	1.0	1.0
	Staff, admissions*	1.0	1.0
	Staff*	0.7	0.7
Therapy	Rehab director	1.0	1.0
	Physical therapist*	0.5	0.5
	Physical therapy assistant*	0.3	0.5
	Occupational therapists*	1.0	1.0
	COTA*	0.7	0.8
	Speech therapist*	0.3	0.4
	Total	**94.4**	**96.1**

NOTE: 1.0 FTE works 1,896 hours per year
* = hourly employee

	2014	2013	2012	2011
Patient days				
Medicare	8,840	8,723	8,690	8,657
Medicaid	22,468	21,858	21,278	20,780
Self-pay	4,420	4,670	4,960	5,140
Other	1,105	1,106	1,530	1,357
Total	**36,833**	**36,357**	**36,458**	**35,934**
Annual occupancy	95.2%	94.0%	94.2%	92.9%
Resident deaths	24	28	27	23
Ancillary services (RVU)				
PT treatments	4,592.00	4,620.20	4,320.00	4,734.50
OT treatments	7,269.60	7,023.00	6,530.00	6,938.00
ST treatments	603.20	580.00	566.40	610.20
Total	**12,464.80**	**12,223.20**	**11,416.40**	**12,282.70**

TABLE 7.4
Operational Statistics by Year

NOTE: 1 RVU = 15-minute service unit

Revenue 2015 Budget	Statement of Operations					
		2014	2013	2012	2011	2010
	Room and board					
	Skilled care					
4,135,329	Medicare Part A	3,977,963	3,820,494	3,820,494	3,724,383	3,650,292
215,383	Commercial	202,582	225,230	210,494	236,191	190,393

TABLE 7.5
Statement of Operations for the 12-Month Period Ending December 31, 2010–2014, and the 2015 Budget ($)

(continued)

TABLE 7.5

Statement of Operations for the 12-Month Period Ending December 31, 2010–2014, and the 2015 Budget ($) (continued)

	Statement of Operations					
Revenue						
2015 Budget		**2014**	**2013**	**2012**	**2011**	**2010**
	Intermediate care					
3,816,373	Medicaid	4,156,604	4,198,356	4,145,291	3,953,282	3,640,439
1,745,292	Self-pay	1,325,988	1,839,202	1,820,394	2,134,203	2,340,203
97,292	VA	92,083	92,363	90,383	189,243	83,405
139,292	Private insurance	97,607	45,393	23,040	21,450	18,450
10,148,961	Total room and board	9,852,827	10,221,038	10,110,096	10,258,752	9,923,182
	Ancillary revenue					
	Skilled care					
834,282	Medicare Parts A and B	795,593	790,373	713,282	702,393	650,393
54,303	Commercial	38,675	39,294	60,393	50,383	47,293
	Intermediate care					
18,373	Medicaid	19,547	14,292	13,258	16,393	18,363
0	Other	0	0	0	0	200
906,958	Total ancillary revenue	853,815	843,959	786,933	769,169	716,249
	Other revenue					
21,494	Interest	18,417	13,292	15,202	16,729	18,560
3,200	Miscellaneous	3,683	3,125	5,403	6,230	3,720
24,694	Total other revenue	22,100	16,417	20,605	22,959	22,280
11,080,613	**Total revenue**	10,728,742	11,081,414	10,917,634	11,050,880	10,661,711
(315,230)	Less provider tax	(313,081)	(343,560)	(313,596)	(302,383)	342,474
(3,129,492)	Less ancillary contractual allowances	(3,057,067)	(3,100,867)	(2,948,202)	(3,000,272)	(2,947,353)
7,635,891	**Total net revenue**	7,358,594	7,636,987	7,655,836	7,748,225	8,056,832
Expenses						
2015 Budget		**2014**	**2013**	**2012**	**2011**	**2010**
	Salaries					
1,790,400	Nursing	1,789,393	1,800,249	1,840,292	1,934,929	1,997,239
560,304	Dietary	556,933	555,002	550,383	480,272	515,388
120,494	Ancillary–PT	103,272	105,230	107,292	107,252	113,282

(continued)

	Statement of Operations					
Expenses						
2015 Budget		**2014**	**2013**	**2012**	**2011**	**2010**
	Salaries					
65,202	Ancillary–OT	62,701	68,303	64,393	58,303	62,120
24,300	Ancillary–ST	22,130	20,130	25,303	27,393	25,303
145,892	Ancillary–RT	140,155	130,202	120,303	127,303	136,303
108,202	Housekeeping	104,383	110,393	131,303	130,292	130,282
135,200	Administration	131,340	141,200	178,202	204,393	180,292
109,303	Social services	104,838	103,292	103,202	103,684	103,606
82,340	Recreation	79,362	80,350	78,383	74,902	78,393
75,300	Physician services	73,278	70,282	82,345	88,202	67,393
60,203	Laundry	58,964	68,002	78,393	88,303	98,303
60,392	Maintenance	55,282	65,303	62,010	60,292	61,202
3,337,532	**Total salaries**	**3,282,031**	**3,317,938**	**3,421,804**	**3,485,520**	**3,569,106**
1,134,761	Benefits, all	956,838	995,381	1,094,977	1,219,932	1,284,878
4,472,293	**Total salaries and benefits**	**4,238,869**	**4,313,319**	**4,516,781**	**4,705,452**	**4,853,984**
	Admin and general	**CY**	**CY-1**	**CY-2**	**CY-3**	**CY-4**
50,000	Accounting fees	60,000	60,000	70,000	80,000	80,000
30,200	Telephone	33,799	34,292	35,292	35,920	36,303
33,000	Insurance–general	30,319	29,200	29,500	34,290	40,202
17,500	Payroll services	18,228	18,200	18,400	16,393	16,300
16,200	MIS management	16,415	16,000	16,000	15,300	15,100
12,500	Dues and licenses	13,054	14,303	13,500	17,202	13,200
10,500	Office supplies	10,424	8,939	7,830	5,920	4,320
8,500	Postage	9,379	9,100	9,320	8,983	7,839
8,000	Legal	8,000	12,503	17,394	12,302	14,393
7,893	Auto	7,893	7,893	7,893	7,893	7,893
5,000	Advertising	6,000	6,000	5,780	5,500	4,000
2,000	Misc. bank charges	3,800	2,000	2,560	2,830	3,210
4,500	Admin equipment rental	4,785	5,640	5,500	4,950	4,640
5,000	Other professional fees	8,979	3,502	3,012	2,640	29,456
1,200	Printing and publishing	1,489	1,648	1,102	1,100	867
211,993	**Total admin and general**	**232,564**	**229,220**	**243,083**	**251,223**	**277,723**

TABLE 7.5

Statement of Operations for the 12-Month Period Ending December 31, 2010–2014, and the 2015 Budget ($) (continued)

(continued)

Expenses 2015 Budget	Statement of Operations					
		2014	2013	2012	2011	2010
	Other operating expenses					
25,300	Maintenance supplies	24,010	22,310	22,740	21,640	20,765
60,383	Maintenance repairs	50,880	34,272	23,784	24,450	26,780
220,450	Utilities–all	219,383	240,120	250,123	250,282	260,383
21,340	Oxygen services	20,175	18,393	17,202	14,383	18,303
277,500	Food	267,039	254,499	255,206	244,351	242,993
200,450	General supplies	202,364	190,303	183,484	178,202	178,202
31,500	Laboratory services	28,511	32,404	28,400	23,450	287,340
210,494	Pharmacy services	207,494	215,450	212,340	215,202	225,202
10,000	Imaging services	11,003	13,204	15,202	11,023	9,303
64,897	Medical equipment rental	64,897	64,897	64,897	60,200	60,200
920,000	Capital lease	900,000	900,000	900,000	900,000	900,000
200,400	Depreciation–all	204,783	205,294	210,494	211,474	211,574
2,242,714	**Total other operating**	**2,202,553**	**2,193,159**	**2,185,884**	**2,156,668**	**2,443,055**
	Nonoperating expenses					
650,000	Management fee	600,000	750,000	550,000	500,000	400,000
4,000	Bad debt	6,600	6,000	5,325	5,270	3,120
654,000	**Total nonoperating**	**606,600**	**756,000**	**555,325**	**505,270**	**403,120**
7,581,000	**Total expenses**	**7,280,586**	**7,491,698**	**7,501,073**	**7,618,613**	**7,977,882**
7,635,891	**Total net revenue**	**7,358,594**	**7,636,987**	**7,655,836**	**7,748,225**	**8,056,832**
54,891	Pretax profit (loss)	78,008	145,289	154,763	129,612	78,950
19,212	All taxes	27,303	50,851	54,167	45,364	27,632
35,679	Profit (loss) after taxes	50,705	94,438	100,596	84,248	51,317

(This table can also be found online at ache.org/books/Middleboro.)

	2014	2013	2012	2011
Assets				
Current				
Cash, operating	3,989,694	3,623,583	3,056,894	2,745,020
Cash, restricted	396,844	382,374	295,750	340,163
Patient trust cash	22,919	24,900	23,491	21,403
Total cash	**4,409,457**	**4,030,857**	**3,376,135**	**3,106,586**
Accounts receivable–net	2,083,242	2,156,393	2,134,265	1,990,237
Inventory	36,404	30,340	22,360	19,372
Prepaid expenses	50,494	45,202	37,345	39,202
Total current assets	**6,579,597**	**6,262,792**	**5,570,105**	**5,155,397**
Plant, property, and equipment (PPE)				
Building, land, and improvements	814,300	795,756	690,202	680,272
Fixed and leasehold fixed equipment	156,303	155,302	155,506	180,383
Furniture and other equipment	1,082,011	995,292	990,385	994,283
Automobile	7,227	14,454	21,681	28,908
Total PPE	**2,059,841**	**1,960,804**	**1,857,774**	**1,883,846**
Less accumulated depreciation	1,246,294	1,041,511	836,217	625,723
Net PPE	813,547	919,293	1,021,557	1,258,123
Other assets				
Security deposits	11,565	9,450	10,474	12,570
Total assets	**7,404,709**	**7,191,535**	**6,602,136**	**6,426,090**
Liabilities and net assets				
Current liabilities				
Accounts payable	1,847,294	1,945,292	1,638,294	1,400,230

TABLE 7.6

Balance Sheet as of December 31 ($)

(continued)

	2014	2013	2012	2011
Accrued expenses	635,640	685,205	690,283	695,304
Patient trust liability	22,919	24,900	23,491	21,403
Accrued interest	9,371	9,145	8,628	8,120
Total current liabilities	**2,515,224**	**2,664,542**	**2,360,696**	**2,125,057**
Long-term liabilities				
Deferred lease obligations	2,541,464	2,734,820	3,028,349	3,450,203
Due to (from) Medicaid	(198,872)	(106,392)	(154,292)	(254,981)
Notes payable	874,260	550,393	525,404	503,282
Line of credit	651,026	655,230	230,450	201,494
Total long-term liabilities	**3,867,878**	**3,710,169**	**3,629,911**	**3,899,998**
Total liabilities	**6,383,102**	**6,374,711**	**5,990,607**	**6,025,055**
Net assets–owners equity	**1,021,607**	**816,824**	**611,529**	**401,035**
Liabilities + net assets	**7,404,709**	**7,191,535**	**6,602,136**	**6,426,090**

(This table can also be found online at ache.org/books/Middleboro.)

Measure	Jasper Gardens	State Average
Overall rating (1 = lowest, 5 = highest)	3	
Health inspections—number of deficiencies	6	0–36
Nursing home staffing (1 = lowest, 5 = highest)	2	
Total number of licensed nurse staff hours per resident per day	1 hr 27 min	
RN hours per resident per day	42 min	
LPN/LVN hours per resident per day	45 min	
Certified nursing assistant hours per resident per day	2 hrs 10 min	

(continued)

Measure	Jasper Gardens	State Average
Quality measures—Overall (1 = lowest, 5 = highest)	5	
Percent of long-stay residents who were given influenza vaccination during the flu season	100	94
Percent of long-stay residents who were assessed and given pneumococcal vaccination	82	95
Percent of long-stay residents whose need for help with daily activities has increased	13	17
Percent of long-stay residents who have moderate to severe pain	2	4
Percent of high-risk long-stay residents who have pressure sores	4	11
Percent of low-risk long-stay residents who have pressure sores	0	5
Percent of long-stay residents who were physically restrained	0	2
Percent of long-stay residents who are more depressed and anxious	13	18
Percent of low-risk long-stay residents who lose control of their bowels or bladder	40	55
Percent of long-stay residents who have/had a catheter inserted and left in their bladder	3	8
Percent of long-stay residents who spend most of their time in bed or in a chair	1	4
Percent of long-stay residents whose ability to move about in and around their room got worse	9	15
Percent of long-stay residents who had a urinary tract infection	4	8
Percent of long-stay residents who lose too much weight	6	10
Percent of short-stay residents given influenza vaccination during the flu season	97	85

TABLE 7.7
CMS Quality Measures as of December 31, 2014
(continued)

(continued)

Measure	Jasper Gardens	State Average
Percent of short-stay residents who were assessed and given pneumococcal vaccination	97	89
Percent of short-stay residents who have delirium	0	2
Percent of short-stay residents who had moderate to severe pain	36	30
Percent of short-stay residents who have pressure sores	6	12
Fire safety inspections—number of deficiencies	2	0–13
Formal complaints	0	2

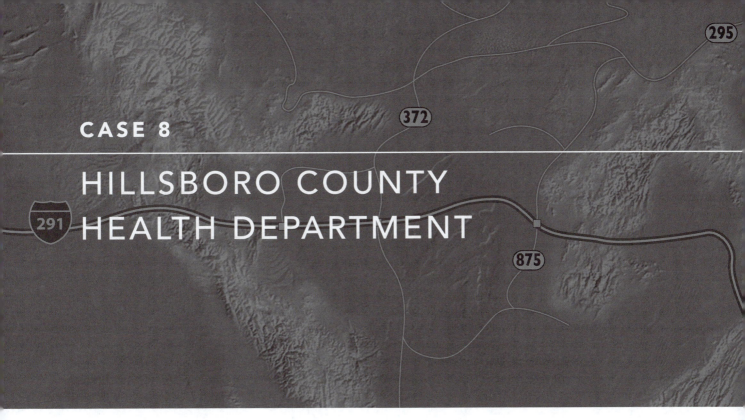

HILLSBORO COUNTY HEALTH DEPARTMENT

The Hillsboro County Health Department (HCHD) was established in 1946. It is a municipal department in the county's government, and it receives all of its funding from Hillsboro County and federal and state grants. Its main offices are in Middleboro. The department is accountable to the Hillsboro County Commissioners. The HCHD also provides oversight of Manorhaven, a 110-bed, county-owned, long-term care facility in Middleboro.

MISSION AND VISION

HCHD's website lists its mission and vision statements as follows:

> To improve the health of individuals, families, and the community through disease prevention, health promotion, and programs to mitigate environmental threats to health and well-being.

> We want Hillsboro County to be a healthy community compared to our state and region. To accomplish this, we are concerned about access to quality healthcare services and an environment free of threats to the public's health.

Hillsboro County Board of Health provides policy guidance. This independent board is appointed by the county commissioners. It was created by statute to identify public health issues and concerns and provide programmatic advice. Members serve five-year terms and can be reappointed. The board is a member of the National Association of Local Boards of Health. Current members include the following:

Name	Profession	Board Role	Term Expires
T. Taylor, DO	Surgeon, Webster Hospital	Chair	2015
M. Foxx, DO, MPH	Physician Care Services	Vice chair	2018
J. Snow	Director, HCHD	Secretary	Ex officio
R. Samuels, MD	Pediatrician, Medical Associates		2016
H. Vosper, RN	Retired		2017
C. Newfields, RN	HC Home Health Agency		2017
J. Masterman, RN, MBA	CEO, Webster Hospital		2015
J. Stock	Middleboro Community Hospital		2019
M. Fudge	School nurse, Middleboro High School		2016
TBD	Community representative		Vacant
TBD	Community representative		Vacant
P. Magnet, DO, MPH	HCHD		Ex officio

The Board of Health's 2014 annual report included the recently revised state guidelines for physical activity in K–12 public schools. The board is considering using these recommendations to help community leaders establish locally supported "Action for Healthy Kids" programs. At least three members of the board advocate adopting these guidelines as a public health priority for 2015–2016.

FUNCTIONAL RESPONSIBILITIES

HCHD collects, disseminates, and monitors health status information as part of its effort to identify physical and environmental health issues. It also assesses the accessibility, effectiveness, and quality of select health services. The department also serves as the county's public health advocate. It defines public health priorities and needs and relies on evidence-based practice to promote, prevent, and improve physical, mental, and environmental health and well-being. Services are provided directly or through grants to area health agencies that carry out the core functions of public health and the essential public health services as defined by the state and the US Centers for Disease Control and Prevention (CDC). The department also studies and reports health problems and hazards using epidemiology. Furthermore, it enforces laws and regulations that protect physical, mental, and environmental health and ensure safety.

Manorhaven is a 110-bed long-term care facility owned and operated by the county. Its administrator reports directly to the HCHD director. Manorhaven is financially independent from the HCHD, but it uses select administrative services (e.g., payroll, human resources) provided by the county. Manorhaven is a distinct line item (i.e., revenue and expense) in the county budget. The administrator of Manorhaven is appointed by the county commissioners based on recommendation of HCHD's director.

ORGANIZATION AND MANAGEMENT

The director of the Hillsboro County Health Department is John Snow. He is responsible for the health of residents in Hillsboro County. He has served in this capacity for 11 years and has been employed by this department for 17 years. He is an appointee of the county, based on a recommendation from the Board of Health, and he serves at the pleasure of the county commissioners. He is a merit-based political appointee and not covered by the county civil service system. Snow holds an undergraduate degree in biology from State University and earned his master of public health at a leading midwestern university. He frequently attends the annual meeting of the American Public Health Association and is on state and national task forces involved with developing a competent public health workforce for the next several decades. He also serves as vice president of the state's Public Health Association and is recognized as the leading spokesperson for public health in nonmetropolitan areas in the state. He has frequently testified before the Committee on Public Health sponsored by the governor and endorsed by the state legislature. As the county health officer, Snow has the responsibility to enforce all state and local regulations, including the ability to fine violators.

When interviewed, Snow said he was concerned that the public health challenges and agenda in Hillsboro County continue to grow, but the funding base continues to shrink. While he indicated total understanding of the need to cut the county's appropriation for public health, he mentioned that some other sources have also cut back. "Some of our larger grants may actually be cancelled in the next one to three years." He indicated that the department has had to cut the work hours of some employees but overall has not had to dismiss any workers. "Any reduction to our workforce has been based on attrition related to retirement or voluntary action." As needed, Candice McCory (Disease Prevention Division) serves as the deputy director of this department.

OFFICE OF THE DIRECTOR

Snow also commented on the aging of his personnel. "I am concerned that within five years, more than one-third of our workers will be eligible for retirement." It has always been difficult to attract qualified workers, especially in environmental health services.

Special challenges include HCHD's unique relationship with Manorhaven. Although Manorhaven has its own separate budget approved by the county commissioners, county regulations hold HCHD responsible for any financial losses. "While this has not been a problem, we are concerned about the future." State Medicaid rates are such that Manorhaven faces an uncertain financial future. It should be noted that 15 years ago, the health department had to cover an $84,000 shortfall in Manorhaven's budget. To maintain oversight, Snow meets quarterly with Manorhaven's management team to review its financial performance. This arrangement between Manorhaven and HCHD was established in 1984 based on the recommendations of a blue-ribbon commission to increase the efficiency of local and county government.

Snow indicated that he felt Hillsboro County's new website has significantly extended the reach and reputation of the health department. He also noted that the continued success of this approach might limit the need for the publication of so many printed annual reports and consumer information sheets.

Five years ago, using federal demonstration grant resources, HCHD began sponsoring two primary care clinics in rural Carterville and Harris City. Other sponsors include Webster Hospital. Each clinic is a 501(c)3 nonprofit organization with a local board of directors. Using space donated by the towns, Rural Clinics, Inc., provides the services of a primary care physician and nurse practitioner. Each clinic is open 10:00 a.m. to 3:00 p.m., Monday through Saturday.

The senior staff of HCHD meets every two weeks to review plans and accomplishments. At these meetings, budget variances are discussed and plans are reviewed for the next 30 to 60 days. Before developing the budget request to the county commissioners, the management team meets with its counterparts in the state Department of Public Health to best estimate state support for county public health programs.

Six years ago, the state Department of Public Health employed a professional liaison in Washington, DC, to monitor and inform the state (and counties) of available federal grants related to their public health missions. The state has indicated that counties will need to contribute to this effort when the existing contract expires in 2016. Snow indicated that this Washington liaison service has led to the county's public health needs being "first in the nation" when grant funding is made available.

This office is also responsible for Health Impact Assessments in accordance with CDC and World Health Organization guidelines. Over the past three years the department has participated in assessments involving municipal transportation systems and land use.

ADMINISTRATIVE SERVICES DIVISION

This division provides management, financial, and administrative support to the entire agency, including grant review and oversight. It is responsible for the preparation and management of the department's budget and staffing plans. The department also retains the part-time services of Dr. Page Magnet, DO, MPH, as the county's health officer and a medical examiner. Jimmy Pagget is the director of this division. He has held this position for 27 years. Prior to his appointment with the health department, he was a senior analyst with the state Department of Revenue Administration. Dr. Magnet meets quarterly with the designated health officers of each of the communities located in Hillsboro County. By statute, each incorporated city and town must designate a health officer to coordinate local services and needs with the county health department. Current health officers are as follows:

City or Town	Name	Occupation
Boalsburg	S. Fistru	Physician, general practice*
Carterville	S. Burns	Deputy chief, Carterville Fire and EMS
Harris City	A. Adams	Physician, general practice*
Jasper	M. Spark	Chief, Jasper Volunteer Fire Department
Middleboro	B. Shovel	Director, Public Works
Mifflenville	B. Fufe	Deputy mayor*
Minortown	I. Kelly	Physician, general practice*
Statesville	M. Clark-Adams	Nurse, retired

*Receives a stipend from city or town less than $1,000 per year to cover time and expenses

Pagget commented on a number of important points and emphasized Snow's perspectives on the department's budget. "While I am grateful that a significant portion of our financial support comes from grants and contracts, they create a vulnerability and potential volatility. Without this support, we could not fulfill our mission." He also mentioned that the State Public Employees Union had recently signed a five-year contract with salary increases of 2 to 3 percent per year and no increases in benefit coverage. Beginning next year, the state's contribution for health and dental insurance is frozen at its current rate and employees will be required to contribute to the cost of their own health insurance. Employees who opt out of the health insurance benefit will receive $4,000. Also an additional week's vacation will be granted to employees with more than 20 years of service. He also indicated that the state and union continue to discuss employee pensions. Currently, workers do not contribute to the state retirement plan, and the state retirement plan is an unfunded liability. The county identifies this as a significant issue.

This division is administratively responsible for all grants and contracts. For grants that allow indirect cost recovery, the division has a 3 percent negotiated indirect cost rate with the US Department of Health and Human Services and the US Environmental Protection Agency. The department receives no indirect reimbursement from state grants and private foundations. When the department awards grants and contracts, it makes no allowances for indirect costs. Only direct costs are covered.

Currently, the HCHD's budget is responsible for facility maintenance and utilities. When a unit of the department is located in a privately owned facility, the department is not responsible for building rental or lease expenses. These costs are covered directly in the facility budget of the county. Each unit in the HCHD has an equipment budget that covers the acquisition and maintenance of all office equipment, including computers. A department-wide committee chaired by Pagget prioritizes and coordinates the acquisition of all equipment, including computers and software. The supplies budget covers office supplies and work-related travel.

ENVIRONMENTAL HEALTH DIVISION

Sally Brownell directs this division. She holds a master of science in environmental health from State University and is a registered environmental health specialist (REHS). She joined the department 18 months ago, having served in a similar position in a western state. Brownell is also a member of the county's HAZMAT team. Her division is responsible for:

- Arboviral program

- Campgrounds (licensure and inspection)

- Emergency preparedness

- Food service sanitation (licensure and inspection)

- Health facility inspection

- Lead paint abatement

- Mosquito and tick control

◆   Public swimming pools

◆   Rabies control

◆   Radon control

◆   Safe water drinking

◆   Sewage treatment—private

The environmental health division maintains multiple contractual relationships with independent laboratories and the state public health laboratory for the provision of laboratory services. Note that the state's Department of Environmental Services performs air quality surveillance.

Brownell states, "Each year's budget requires us to adjust to our level of support. For example, the division has had to prioritize its inspections. Our current policy is that if an establishment that engages in food preparation has passed inspection without any conditions for four consecutive years, the department can (if needed) waive the fifth-year inspection."

Specific areas were noted as significant concerns. This past year, the lead control program suffered from a change in leadership and its coverage for home inspections was limited. The housing stock, especially in the northern part of the county, needs increased attention given its age, the prevalence of lead paint, and the resettlement of refugees and immigrants who have limited English proficiency. When secondary prevention measures are implemented, children regularly present with elevated blood lead levels. If not addressed, these elevated blood levels can eventually negatively affect cognitive development and school performance, thus leading to increased social costs. Unless the department is better able to demonstrate to the state its need for this program, it may face curtailment or elimination.

Another housing-related issue in the community has been bedbug infestations in the low-income districts of the county. This environmental issue is a nuisance that can be attributed to absentee landlords, poor-quality living conditions, social determinants of health, and diverse populations with limited English proficiency. This division is trying to educate the occupants of these units about preventive measures and connect them with social service agencies that can provide better-quality furniture.

Since the banning of DDT spraying 35 years ago, mosquito control remains an issue. State funding has ceased for mosquito surveillance in the county. As a result, under the direction of this division, community volunteers are used to assist in mosquito control programs countywide as a cost-effective approach to conduct surveillance for the presence of mosquito-borne diseases, such as West Nile virus and Eastern equine encephalitis.

EPA has identified one hazardous waste site in the county. In the 1950s and 1960s the JM Asbestos Company inadvertently contaminated the soil, groundwater, and the

Swift River that runs through the county. The extent of the environmental contamination and the resultant health effects on the employees of the company and their families—as well as local residents who lived within a five-mile radius of the company and those who fished downstream from the plant—qualified this area to be declared a Superfund site. This division is working with the EPA and the Agency for Toxic Substances and Disease Registry (ATSDR) to conduct a public health assessment.

Recently the department requested that the ATSDR provide a health consultation to identify and assess the site owned by Carlstead Rayon. Preliminary studies indicate that Carlstead Rayon will be designated a hazardous waste site. Carlstead Rayon has indicated that if this occurs it may need to abandon its current facility and leave the county. Brownell has also testified before the legislature regarding the following bills:

◆   HB 2701 would eliminate water fluoridation. This bill is being amended to require a warning to property owners served by municipal water systems that their water supply is fluoridated. This warning would be included in the quarterly water bill.

◆   HB 2405 would allow communities to impose a moratorium on refugee resettlement in the county.

COMMUNITY HEALTH PROMOTION DIVISION

Russell Martin directs this division. He has held this position for nine years. His credentials include a master's of public health from a leading midwestern university and more than 10 years' experience in a similar position with the state Department of Public Health. He is scheduled to retire within the next two years. This division contracts with area health providers to address some of the following responsibilities:

◆   Vision screening

◆   Hearing screening

◆   Tobacco control

◆   School health (including oral health)

◆   Substance abuse prevention

◆   Adult health promotion

Martin also serves on the regional and state Emergency Preparedness Task Force.

This division maintains an active adult health and osteoporosis prevention and screening program. It frequently sponsors programs with the local chapter of AARP, Red

Cross, and Rural Clinics, Inc. Clinics and screening programs are held countywide, including at Manorhaven. Health promotion seminars, workshops, and fairs are also held in every public school in the county. Three times a year the HCHD, with one or more corporate sponsors, organizes 5k road races to call attention to health promotion and obesity.

The tobacco control program includes the enforcement of state and county regulation involving smoking in public and in any licensed organization, such as restaurants, barbershops, and so on. Aside from holding smoking cessation classes quarterly, this division provides literature at numerous health fairs throughout the county.

The oral health program currently screens elementary school children each year for dental caries. Two dental hygienists run the program in this division and conduct oral screenings and cleanings and apply dental sealants. Two dentists, based in the community, each volunteer once per week during the school year to conduct minor procedures, such as extractions. The program is administered via a mobile dental van that travels to each of the six elementary schools. The Kiwanis Club donated the mobile dental van, which is in need of major repairs and will cost approximately $300,000 to replace.

Within the last six months the Jasper Regional Educational Cooperative approached the department with the plan to contract with the department for all staff and services related to school health. Under this plan this cooperative school board would transfer all current school health funding to the department and sign a five-year renewable contract for expanded services. This plan is under active review. Martin indicated that grant funds might be available to expand current services, especially in health behavior, such as a hand washing campaign in schools and all licensed educational and healthcare facilities.

Snow has recently asked Martin to draft the department's response to a letter printed in the local paper. The letter advocated banning sugary drinks in all public schools and adopting healthy vending policies. The leader of a local coalition of concerned parents and nurses signed the letter.

DISEASE PREVENTION DIVISION

Candice McCory, RN, MS, has directed this division for 27 years. She holds an undergraduate degree in nursing and an advanced certificate in epidemiology from State University. Her division provides direct services and services via contracts with area health agencies. This division is responsible for:

◆ Breast and cervical cancer screening

◆ Communicable disease control including case investigations

◆ Family planning education and services

◆ Healthy eating

◆   HIV/AIDS counseling and testing

◆   Immunization planning and clinics

◆   STD diagnosis and treatment referrals

◆   Women, Infants, and Children (WIC) programs

When interviewed, McCory said her division "had the highest level of professionalism and productivity. I am especially proud of our workers and what we have accomplished with limited resources." She also mentioned that her division managed a countywide immunization and dental health program. "We are especially fortunate that so many area dentists volunteer their time to provide indigent dental care, especially in the rural parts of our county." McCory expressed specific concerns about rural women. "Women's health is a significant issue in this county, especially in our rural communities. Needs and issues just aren't identified, they are addressed. In response to this concern, we now either hold or sponsor family planning clinics throughout the county frequently, in conjunction with programs and services provided under the WIC program." She indicated that her attempts to organize women's health outreach programs by each hospital and other health providers has had limited success. "Of all the area providers, the Hillsboro County Home Health Agency's Community Health Division is the most responsive to our needs."

Recently, state funding for STD screening, including HIV/AIDS counseling, has been cut. As a result, the public health specialist I position was eliminated. Prior to the termination of this position, the standardized mortality ratio for HIV/AIDS in the county was greater than 1.0.

Last month, McCory was asked to develop recommendations with a budget to address expanding the adult immunization services provided by the department. With the availability of influenza immunization in area pharmacies, perhaps the health department should no longer provide this service and instead focus on other immunization programs, such as shingles vaccines for the population older than age 60.

ISSUES AND CONCERNS

The governor has announced a statewide task force on public health to report back in 2016. The task force, composed of statewide business and civic leaders, is charged with examining whether regional health departments are more economical than county-specific ones. Under their tentative plan, regional health departments covering between 1 and 1.5 million lives would be organized under the direct control of the state Department of Public Health. Individual counties would be billed for their share of the cost. The statewide chapter of county commissioners opposes this plan, saying it removes local control but requires local taxes to support statewide programs.

Brownell, Martin, and McCory have formally requested that the HCHD reconsider its current organizational structure. They have asked that consultants be hired to address three questions.

1. Should we be organized into three divisions? If so, what should those divisions have as their primary responsibilities? If not, how should we be organized?

2. Should the administrative services division be separate or folded into the office of the director and the program-oriented divisions?

3. What services and programs can and should we contract to other health agencies, such as area hospitals and the Hillsboro County Home Health Agency?

Snow has indicated that he will discuss these questions with the county commissioners and report back whether financial support for consulting services will be part of the department's annual budget request.

A recent editorial in the local newspaper questioned whether the department was prepared to address public health issues such as a flu epidemic. Also, the State Board of Health has recommended that small county departments, such as HCHD, must either expand their services or contract with other local healthcare agencies to create regional (local) health departments. The department is currently considering the issues and alternatives.

Note that the HCHD is charged with local responsibility for implementing a newly revised statewide Medicaid waiver under section 1915 (c). This Home and Community-based Services waiver allows Medicaid to cover the expenses of community-based homes for special population (e.g., patients with intellectual and development disabilities) and screen all Medicaid-eligible patients before they are admitted to a residential long-term care facility. Under the revised plan, any individual who is Medicaid-eligible and can be cared for at home will be denied admission into a nursing home.

It should be noted that in the past five years, the state has twice been found to be in violation of the Supreme Court Olmstead decision of 1999, which held that segregating people with disabilities is a violation of the Americans with Disabilities Act and public entities must provide community-based services to people with disabilities.

Approximately 40 percent of the resources used to support public health programs in Hillsboro County are from grants and contracts. According to Snow, "This makes us especially vulnerable to changes in funding at the federal, state, and local levels. Unless our county's economy improves, I am sure it will not approve increasing expenditures for public health."

Snow recently returned from a national meeting involving the National Public Health Performance Standards Program and indicated that the HCHD should become significantly more engaged with this national program. He has requested that the senior staff provide a recommendation to him and the Board of Health whether the HCHD should seek national accreditation and whether it currently meets or can meet the national standards for a local health department. "It appears that the marginal benefits associated with accreditation far exceed its marginal costs."

Snow continues his conversations with the county commissioners about emergency preparedness. Currently, city and town fire, police, and ambulance services provide the leadership for countywide emergency preparedness. Annually, the existing 24-member emergency preparedness committee is obligated to provide the county commissioners a status report describing the county's current readiness to address large-scale emergencies and recommendations for action. The county still has not achieved communication system integration involving all its first responders. Snow continues to suggest that the committee be made responsible to the county Board of Health. Currently, no changes are anticipated.

Currently, the state contributes 50 percent of funding for the Medicaid program. The state has indicated that, given anticipated Medicaid cost increases, it will either need to increase statewide taxes or require counties to contribute 10 to 25 percent of the Medicaid expenditures in their county. Under one of their plans, the state Medicaid program would pay 80 percent of allowable charges based on the statewide fee schedule and the county would pay the remaining 20 percent. According to Snow, such a program would bankrupt public health's ability to fulfill its mission.

In keeping with its population growth, the city of Jasper continues to expand its municipal water and sewage system. Fifteen years ago, town water and sewer systems covered 12 percent of city property. Today, these systems cover 54 percent. The city estimates that 88 percent of the households in Jasper will be serviced with town water and sewer within six years. The city has, however, recently declared a moratorium on adding fluoridation to town water systems, effective July 2015. In 2011, the Jasper City Council received a petition with 6,100 signatures against fluoridation. This led to the council's original decision against fluoridation. Two current members of the Jasper City Council—Kip and Simpson—have continued to vote against fluoridation.

Nationally the number of cases of community-acquired MRSA (methicillin-resistant Staphylococcus aureus) has attracted local concern. Snow has asked the senior staff for policy recommendations.

	2004	2009	2014
Annual licensed food establishments	523	745	712
Routine inspections conducted	1,320	956	1,258
Reinspections conducted	237	177	101
Complaint investigations conducted	163	167	153
Temporary food stand inspections	102	312	228
Food certification classes	9	23	14
Potable water supply			
Water well permits issued	45	56	68
Water wells installed	15	32	43
New water well inspections	20	28	42
Complaint investigations conducted	12	18	2
Private onsite wastewater disposal			
System permits issued	152	177	187
Systems installed	98	101	169
System inspections	164	130	197
Complaint investigations conducted	21	14	24
Lead hazards removal			
Environmental assessments	60	77	146
Homes mitigated	15	85	174
Other			
Indoor tanning establishment inspections	15	24	27
Body art establishment inspections	4	5	7

TABLE 8.1
Environmental
Health Statistics

(continued)

TABLE 8.1
Environmental
Health Statistics
(continued)

	2004	2009	2014
Camp (summer) inspections	59	58	40
Health facility inspections	12	18	19
Public swimming pool inspections	10	11	11
Rabies control investigations	5	8	16
Radon control inspections	12	14	13
Vector control public contacts	245	201	225
Vector control inspections	80	133	157

	2004	2009	2014
Adult health program			
Health clinics conducted	21	18	20
Clients seen	1,405	1,466	1,177
Vision screening clients	459	689	544
Hearing screening clients	857	818	801
Substance abuse pamphlets distributed	1,350	1,400	14,000
Health promotion presentations			
Community programs given	34	80	99
Community program attendees	978	1,326	1,277
School health program presentations	159	156	201
School health program attendees	3,948	3,648	4,106
Health fairs attended	16	14	16
Osteoporosis prevention and screening			
Women screened	224	203	190
Tobacco-free community programs			
Smoking cessation program enrollees	112	167	180
Program classes	14	36	27
Smoke-free complaints	64	81	44
Smoke-free inspections	5	3	6
Smoke-free fines assessed	8	3	5

TABLE 8.2
Community Health and Health Promotion Statistics

	2004	2009	2014
Communicable diseases reported			
Giardiasis	5	9	6
Lyme disease	22	9	15
Meningitis (viral)	0	1	0
Salmonellosis	9	14	13
Shigellosis	5	11	3
Tuberculosis	1	3	0
Case investigations (includes STD)	9	6	11
Dental health program			
Examinations	3,277	2,503	2,145
Sealants	509	503	565
Other dental services	3,715	4,129	4,423
Family planning			
Clinics held	4	5	8
Immunizations			
Adult immunization doses administered	3,512	3,823	3,718
Adult immunization clients served	2,546	2,156	2,247
Childhood immunization doses administered	9,213	8,934	8,560
Childhood immunization clients served	3,068	3,312	3,369
H1N1 vaccine doses administered	823	1,201	1,422
Influenza immunization adult doses	434	623	827
Influenza immunization infant/child doses	338	602	801

(continued)

	2004	2009	2014
Sexually transmitted diseases			
Clinic patient encounters	1,856	2,099	2,178
HIV counseling and testing at clinics	892	757	1,002
Chlamydia cases reported	956	1,130	1,268
Gonorrhea cases reported	402	386	406
Syphilis cases reported	0	1	1
Women, Infants, and Children (WIC) program			
Clients certified	5,103	6,022	6,835
Clients attending nutrition classes	3,046	3,156	3,821
Breastfeeding peer counseling contracts	n/a	187	203
High-risk infant visits	87	134	202
Children with elevated blood lead levels	69	51	44
Women's health			
Clients seen	2,056	2,014	2,544

TABLE 8.3
Disease Prevention
Statistics
(continued)

TABLE 8.4
Statement of
Revenue and
Expenses as of
December 31 ($)

	2014	2013	2012
Revenue			
County appropriation/tax levy	2,421,165	2,553,000	2,870,525
Federal grants			
CDC environmental health tracking	8,450	8,450	8,200
EPA—asthma	37,566	35,688	33,903
Oral health	21,705	24,340	27,393
Rural healthcare development	194,204	212,440	215,383
Rural poverty and homelessness	103,440	90,450	85,303
State grants			
County health department development	215,400	200,000	200,000
EMS assistance	121,000	110,000	110,000
EMS preparedness	45,000	45,000	45,000
HIV control and prevention	55,000	55,000	55,000
Immunization	68,445	50,000	50,000
Lead control program	15,787	15,000	12,450
Medicaid oral health	118,407	94,818	56,282
Primary healthcare—demo	234,040	212,494	0
STD control and prevention	83,817	85,000	85,000
Tobacco use	56,818	72,404	86,249
WIC administration	85,000	85,000	85,000
WIC services	357,202	325,493	365,292
Private foundations			
Breast cancer awareness	40,000	30,000	0
Obesity control and prevention	2,175	0	0
Subtotal external grants and contracts	**1,863,456**	**1,751,577**	**1,520,455**

(continued)

	2014	2013	2012	
Licenses and permits				
Food services	6,219	5,740	5,952	
Campgrounds	1,250	1,433	1,340	
Tanning facilities	450	560	0	
Special fees and fines	2,430	3,145	3,767	
Overhead recovery[1]	100,113	125,000	150,300	
Other—misc.	204	612	120	
Subtotal noncounty tax revenue	1,974,122	1,888,067	1,681,934	
Total revenue	**4,395,287**	**4,441,067**	**4,552,459**	
Expenses				
Office of the director				
Salaries and wages	262,969	260,314	256,408	
Benefits	73,631	77,286	71,063	
Supplies	18,540	21,500	20,340	
Equipment	24,660	24,302	12,560	
Utilities[2]	2,422	2,200	2,030	
Marketing and promotion	4,000	4,000	5,000	
Staff development	500	4,000	4,000	
Misc.	2,366	596	856	
Grants to local agencies	4,800	6,800	6,800	
Subtotal	**393,888**	**400,998**	**379,057**	
Administrative services division				
Salaries and wages	523,420	500,200	553,487	
Benefits	157,026	155,062	171,580	
Supplies	84,284	94,563	99,363	

TABLE 8.4
Statement of Revenue and Expenses as of December 31 ($) (continued)

(continued)

	2014	2013	2012
Equipment	4,803	5,234	4,109
Utilities[2]	28,383	26,440	28,304
Marketing and promotion	450	500	500
Staff development	1,000	1,500	2,000
Misc.	200	140	167
Grants to local agencies	0	0	0
Subtotal	**799,566**	**783,639**	**859,510**
Environmental health division			
Salaries and wages	452,320	456,675	446,905
Benefits	135,696	141,569	138,541
Supplies	6,579	6,500	5,356
Equipment	1,039	2,546	2,946
Utilities[2]	37,669	36,122	35,476
Marketing and promotion	3,825	4,024	6,034
Staff development	500	4,000	4,000
Misc.—lab contracts	4,375	3,760	3,700
Misc.	243	201	103
Grants to local agencies	0	0	0
Subtotal	**642,246**	**655,397**	**643,061**
Community health and health promotion			
Salaries and wages	765,744	762,971	735,923
Benefits	222,066	236,521	228,136
Supplies	98,161	103,453	117,506
Equipment	39,445	23,450	12,404
Utilities[2]	22,341	23,460	24,354
Marketing and promotion	4,512	5,500	5,500
Staff development	355	5,000	5,000

(continued)

	2014	2013	2012
Misc.	456	402	450
Grants to local agencies	124,565	135,400	150,220
Subtotal	**1,277,645**	**1,296,157**	**1,279,493**
Personal health and health protection			
Salaries and wages	765,957	780,156	847,233
Benefits	237,447	241,848	262,642
Supplies	103,288	110,393	114,506
Equipment	23,693	12,000	4,500
Utilities[2]	34,552	34,595	30,282
Marketing and promotion	2,300	2,500	2,500
Staff development	1,800	4,800	4,800
Misc.	356	221	498
Grants to local agencies	112,445	118,340	124,303
Subtotal	**1,281,838**	**1,304,853**	**1,391,264**
Total expenses	**4,395,183**	**4,441,045**	**4,552,385**
Excess revenue[3]	104	22	74

TABLE 8.4

Statement of Revenue and Expenses as of December 31 ($) (continued)

NOTES: 1. The amount included in grants to cover overhead. Used to reduce expenses.
2. Total charges for utilities are allocated based on square feet occupied.
3. Excess revenue is returned to the general fund at the end of the fiscal year.

(This table can also be found online at ache.org/books/Middleboro.)

TABLE 8.5

Budget by Source of Funds, 2014 ($)

	Office of the Director	Administrative Services	Environmental Health	Community Health and Health Promotion	Personal Health and Health Protection	Total
Federal grants						
CDC environmental health tracking			8,450			8,450
EPA—asthma			37,566			37,566
Oral health					21,705	21,705
Rural healthcare development	21,000	50,000	80,060	43,144		194,204
Rural poverty and homelessness	18,000			74,800	10,640	103,440
State grants						
County health department development	118,450	950	32,000	32,000	32,000	215,400
EMS assistance				121,000		121,000
EMS preparedness				45,000		45,000
HIV control and prevention				30,000	25,000	55,000
Immunization					68,445	68,445
Lead control program			15,787			15,787
Medicaid oral health					118,407	118,407
Primary healthcare—demo			9,475	224,565		234,040
STD control and prevention					83,817	83,817
Tobacco use				56,818		56,818
WIC administration	25,500	15,600			43,900	85,000
WIC services					357,202	357,202
Private foundations						
Breast cancer awareness				40,000		40,000
Obesity control and prevention				2,175		2,175
Total grants and contracts	182,950	66,550	183,338	669,502	761,116	1,863,456
Other revenue	10,553					10,553
Overhead recovery		100,113				100,113
Total noncounty revenue	193,503	166,663	183,338	669,502	761,116	1,974,122
County tax appropriation	200,385	632,903	458,908	608,143	520,722	2,421,061
Total budget by division	393,888	799,566	642,246	1,277,645	1,281,838	4,395,183
Percent total budget—county funds	50.9%	79.2%	71.5%	47.6%	40.6%	55.1%

(This table can also be found online at ache.org/books/Middleboro.)

TABLE 8.6

Staffing Budget, 2012–2014 ($)

	2014		2013		2012	
Office of the director	FTE	Budgeted Salary	FTE	Budgeted Salary	FTE	Budgeted Salary
Director	1.0	130,174	1.0	130,174	1.0	130,174
Administrative assistant III	1.0	39,262	1.0	38,477	1.0	37,322
Administrative assistant II	0.5	31,348	0.0	30,721	0.0	29,799
Health info tech	0.5	44,560	0.5	43,669	0.5	42,359
Intern	0.5	17,625	0.5	17,273	0.5	16,754
Subtotal	**3.5**	**262,969**	**3.0**	**260,314**	**3.0**	**256,408**
Administrative services						
Deputy director for administration	1.0	92,330	1.0	90,483	1.0	88,674
Public health medical director	0.5	98,517	0.5	98,517	0.5	98,517
Business services officer	1.2	90,315	1.0	73,787	1.0	72,340
Customer service rep II	1.0	53,315	1.0	52,249	1.0	51,204
Administrative services manager	1.0	51,230	2.0	50,205	2.0	49,201
Administrative assistant II	1.0	31,348	1.0	30,721	1.0	30,107
Custodian	2.5	106,365	3.0	104,238	4.0	163,444
Subtotal	**8.2**	**523,420**	**9.5**	**500,200**	**10.5**	**553,487**
Environmental health						
Deputy director for environmental health	1.0	103,233	1.0	101,168	1.0	101,168
Environmental health specialist IV	1.0	54,223	1.0	53,139	1.0	53,139
Environmental health specialist II	4.0	135,056	4.0	132,408	4.0	129,812
Public health specialist II	2.0	128,460	2.0	125,891	2.0	119,598
Administrative assistant II	1.0	31,348	1.0	30,721	1.0	30,107
Administrative assistant I	0.0	0	0.5	13,348	0.5	13,081
Subtotal	**9.0**	**452,320**	**9.5**	**456,675**	**9.5**	**446,905**
Community health and health promotion						
Deputy director for community health	1.0	93,274	1.0	88,610	1.0	86,838
Community health nurse	6.0	379,260	6.0	367,882	6.0	360,525
Public health specialist II	3.0	192,960	3.0	183,312	3.0	179,646
Public health preparedness admin	1.0	86,200	1.3	109,819	1.0	82,752
Administrative assistant I	0.5	14,050	0.5	13,348	1.0	26,163
Subtotal	**11.5**	**765,744**	**11.8**	**762,971**	**12.0**	**735,923**
Personal health and health protection						
Deputy director for personal health	1.0	104,330	1.0	99,114	1.0	97,131
Public health specialist III	2.0	120,068	2.0	114,065	3.0	111,783
Program director for women's health	1.0	84,670	1.0	80,437	1.0	78,828
Public health nurse	5.0	332,115	5.0	315,509	5.0	247,360
Case control investigator	1.0	84,550	1.4	86,173	2.0	162,336
Community services assistant	0.5	24,550	1.5	69,968	2.0	91,425
Administrative assistant II	0.5	15,674	1.0	14,890	2.0	58,370
Subtotal	**11.0**	**765,957**	**12.9**	**780,156**	**16.0**	**847,233**
Total	**43.2**	**2,770,410**	**46.7**	**2,760,315**	**51.0**	**2,839,956**

(This table can also be found online at ache.org/books/Middleboro.)

TABLE 8.7

Special Study: Oral Health Issues and Fluoridation

Percentage of households served by a municipal water system	2014	2009	2004
Boalsburg	0	0	0
Carterville	12	12	10
Harris City	8	4	5
Jasper	54	50	44
Middleboro	74	73	70
Mifflenville	22	24	30
Minortown	5	10	12
Statesville	18	20	9

Percentage of households served by a fluoridated water system	2014	2009	2004
Boalsburg	0	0	0
Carterville	4	4	4
Harris City	0	0	0
Jasper	54	50	44
Middleboro	54	58	56
Mifflenville	22	24	0
Minortown	0	0	0
Statesville	0	10	12

2010 special study of third-grade students by town of residence	Tooth Decay	Untreated Tooth Decay	
Percent of students with			
Boalsburg	43.6	12.9	
Carterville	19.3	14.3	
Harris City	28.2	13.2	
Jasper	23.5	8.1	

(continued)

2010 special study of third-grade students by town of residence	Tooth Decay	Untreated Tooth Decay	
Middleboro	24.9	10.7	
Mifflenville	32.9	15.2	
Minortown	31.4	23.7	
Statesville	29.7	11.4	
2012 special study of dental cleaning by dentist or hygienist			
Last cleaning within _ years*	2 years	5 years	6 or more
Boalsburg	60	15	25
Carterville	56	10	34
Harris City	62	17	21
Jasper	79	10	11
Middleboro	70	14	16
Mifflenville	64	14	22
Minortown	77	10	13
Statesville	56	12	32

NOTE: *Never or Did not know included in 6 years or more

TABLE 8.7
Special Study:
Oral Health Issues
and Fluoridation
(continued)

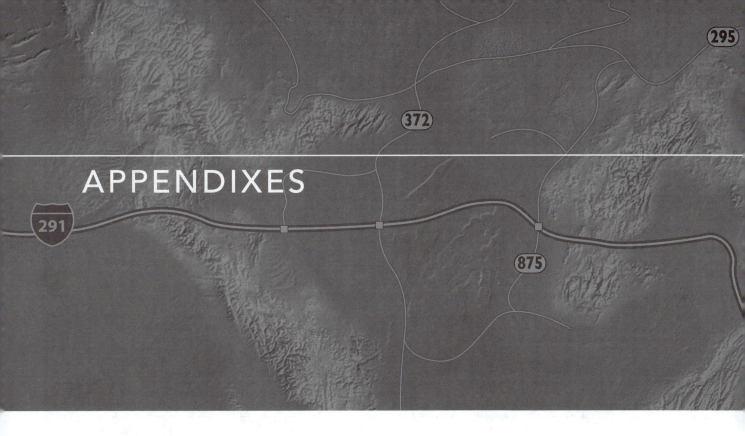

295

372

875

APPENDIXES

Appendixes include supplemental information on Capital City. Although not located in Hillsboro County, Capital City is near Jasper. As stated in the case, Jasper is slowly becoming a commuter town for Capital City; an increasing number of Jasper residents are working in Capital City. The travel time between Jasper and Capital City will be reduced significantly with the opening of the new highway. Capital City also remains the medical referral center for Hillsboro County.

The following appendixes are included:

A.1 Capital City Population: 1989–2014 (This table can also be found online at ache.org/books/Middleboro.)

A.2 Age Profile for Capital City, 2014

A.3 Vital Statistics for Capital City

A.4 Capital City Resident Deaths by Cause of Death

A.5 Capital City Age-Specific Deaths: 2009 and 2014

A.6 CMS Core Measures for Hospitals in Capital City: 2014 Capital City General (CCG) and Osteopathic Medical Center (OMC)

TABLE A.1

Capital City Population: 1989–2014

All Races	1989	1994	1999	2004	2009	2014
Ward I	37,450	39,339	41,249	40,320	41,250	40,293
Ward II	45,204	46,503	47,502	50,395	52,395	50,392
Ward III	18,346	21,340	29,720	31,370	31,595	35,202
Ward IV	9,450	13,268	36,869	38,145	38,200	51,673
Total	110,450	120,450	155,340	160,230	163,440	177,560
White	**1989**	**1994**	**1999**	**2004**	**2009**	**2014**
Ward I	30,070	31,898	28,272	26,646	25,949	19,241
Ward II	40,214	38,987	39,815	42,599	44,057	38,668
Ward III	13,774	17,088	24,590	25,971	25,350	27,212
Ward IV	8,790	12,603	35,867	37,123	35,387	48,936
Total	92,848	100,576	128,544	132,339	130,743	134,057
Black	**1989**	**1994**	**1999**	**2004**	**2009**	**2014**
Ward I	6,524	6,506	11,627	12,096	13,612	19,202
Ward II	4,428	6,927	6,927	6,826	7,218	10,294
Ward III	4,252	3,820	4,368	4,516	5,365	7,067
Ward IV	189	212	379	597	1,590	1,612
Total	15,393	17,465	23,301	24,035	27,785	38,175
Other	**1989**	**1994**	**1999**	**2004**	**2009**	**2014**
Ward I	856	935	1,350	1,578	1,689	1,850
Ward II	562	589	760	970	1,120	1,430
Ward III	320	432	762	883	880	923
Ward IV	471	453	623	425	1,223	1,125
Total	2,209	2,409	3,495	3,856	4,912	5,328

(This table can also be found online at ache.org/books/Middleboro.)

	Total	Under 5	5–14	15–24	25–44	45–64	65–74	75+
Ward I	**40,295**	**2,760**	**5,698**	**5,318**	**12,001**	**8,660**	**3,497**	**2,361**
Male	**19,939**	1,396	2,991	2,692	5,284	4,446	2,133	997
Female	**20,355**	1,364	2,707	2,626	6,717	4,213	1,364	1,364
Ward II	**50,391**	**3,450**	**7,122**	**6,648**	**15,024**	**10,826**	**4,364**	**2,957**
Male	**24,691**	1,728	3,704	3,333	6,543	5,506	2,642	1,235
Female	**25,700**	1,722	3,418	3,315	8,481	5,320	1,722	1,722
Ward III	**35,202**	**2,408**	**4,962**	**4,640**	**10,545**	**7,551**	**3,018**	**2,078**
Male	**16,488**	1,154	2,473	2,226	4,370	3,677	1,764	824
Female	**18,714**	1,254	2,489	2,414	6,175	3,874	1,254	1,254
Ward IV	**51,673**	**3,537**	**7,294**	**6,815**	**15,440**	**11,093**	**4,454**	**3,040**
Male	**24,802**	1,736	3,720	3,348	6,573	5,531	2,654	1,240
Female	**26,869**	1,800	3,574	3,466	8,867	5,562	1,800	1,800
Total	**177,561**	**12,155**	**25,076**	**23,421**	**53,010**	**38,130**	**15,333**	**10,436**
Male	**85,921**	6,014	12,888	11,599	22,770	19,161	9,193	4,296
Female	**91,638**	6,140	12,188	11,821	30,240	18,969	6,140	6,140
% Male	**48.4%**	49.5%	51.4%	49.5%	43.0%	50.3%	60.0%	41.2%
% Female	**51.6%**	50.5%	48.6%	50.5%	57.0%	49.7%	40.0%	58.8%

TABLE A.2
Age Profile for Capital City, 2014

	1989	1994	1999	2004	2009	2014
Live births	1,667	1,723	2,051	2,163	2,257	2,556
Deaths (except fetal)	1,056	1,145	1,398	1,362	1,379	1,456
Infant deaths[1]	25	24	22	21	19	18
Neonatal deaths[2]	14	15	14	14	12	11
Postneonatal deaths[3]	11	9	8	7	7	7
Maternal deaths	2	0	2	3	1	2
Out-of-wedlock births	178	245	315	565	689	890
Marriages	1,125	1,325	1,325	1,433	1,358	1,367

TABLE A.3
Vital Statistics for Capital City

NOTES:
1. Under 1 year
2. Under 28 days
3. 28 days to 11 months

TABLE A.4

Capital City
Resident Deaths by
Cause of Death

Cause of Death	Note	1989	1994	1999	2004	2009	2014
Diseases of the heart	A	268	295	365	361	376	418
Malignant neoplasms	B	210	267	296	298	300	340
Cerebrovascular diseases	C	68	78	84	80	85	96
All accidents	D	60	56	58	50	60	67
Chronic lower respiratory disease	E	49	58	67	60	69	77
Influenza and pneumonia	F	38	39	38	41	30	40
Diabetes mellitus	G	34	30	40	31	34	45
Alzheimer's disease	H	12	16	39	18	30	39
Intentional self-harm/suicide	I	22	35	21	15	17	19
Nephritis, nephrotic syndrome, and nephrosis	J	25	19	28	20	20	25
Septicemia	K	10	18	12	12	20	20
Total leading causes		**796**	**911**	**1,048**	**986**	**1,041**	**1,186**
All deaths		**1,049**	**1,152**	**1,398**	**1,378**	**1,340**	**1,456**

NOTES: ICD codes

A I00-I09, I11, I13, I20-I51
B C00-C97
C I60-I69
D V01-X59, Y85-Y86
E J4-0-J47
F J10-J18
G E10-E14
H G30
I U03,X60-X84, Y87.0
J N00-N07, N17-N19, N25-N27
K A40-A41

Cause of Death	Total	Under 1	1– 4	5– 14	15– 24	25– 44	45– 64	65– 75	75+
Diseases of the heart									
2014	418	0	0	0	0	11	50	139	218
2009	376	0	0	0	0	9	40	101	226
Malignant neoplasms									
2014	340	0	0	2	4	9	15	145	165
2009	300	0	3	4	6	24	41	94	128
Cerebrovascular diseases									
2014	96	0	0	0	0	2	14	33	47
2009	85	0	0	0	0	5	17	26	37
All accidents									
2014	67	3	3	4	16	15	12	5	9
2009	60	6	1	2	13	16	8	3	11
Chronic lower respiratory disease									
2014	77	0	0	0	0	0	21	29	27
2009	69	0	0	0	4	9	18	24	14
Influenza and pneumonia									
2014	40	3	2	0	0	0	2	8	25
2009	40	0	1	0	0	4	4	9	22
Diabetes mellitus									
2014	45	0	0	0	0	4	20	12	9
2009	34	0	0	0	0	5	12	12	5
Alzheimer's disease									
2014	39	0	0	0	0	0	1	10	28
2009	30	0	0	0	0	0	4	9	17
Intentional self-harm									
2014	19	0	1	6	3	3	3	2	1
2009	17	0	0	3	2	3	6	1	2

TABLE A.5

Capital City Age-Specific Deaths: 2009 and 2014

(continued)

Cause of Death	Total	Under 1	1–4	5–14	15–24	25–44	45–64	65–75	75+
Nephritis, nephrotic syndrome, nephrosis									
2014	25	1	0	4	2	4	6	2	6
2009	20	0	1	5	3	1	2	2	6
Septicemia									
2014	20	2	0	0	0	0	6	5	7
2009	20	1	0	2	0	5	4	4	4
Total—listed causes									
2014	1,186	9	6	16	25	48	150	390	542
2009	1,041	7	6	16	28	81	146	285	472
Total—other causes									
2014	270	9	30	19	23	31	43	48	67
2009	338	12	14	7	17	14	42	115	117
Total—all deaths									
2014	1,456	18	36	35	48	79	193	438	609
2009	1,379	19	20	23	45	95	188	400	589

Category	CMS Core Measure	State Benchmark	2014 CCG	2014 OMC
Timely Heart Attack Care	Average number of minutes before outpatient with chest pain or possible heart attack who needed specialized care was transferred to another hospital	1 hr	n/a	n/a
Timely Heart Attack Care	Average number of minutes before outpatients with chest pain or possible heart attack got an ECG	8 min	9 min	5 min
Timely Heart Attack Care	Outpatients with chest pain or possible heart attack who got aspirin within 24 hours of arrival	100%	92%	100%

(continued)

Category	CMS Core Measure	State Benchmark	2014 CCG	2014 OMC
Timely Heart Attack Care	Heart attack patients given PCI within 90 minutes of arrival	94%	99%	98%
Effective Heart Attack Care	Heart attack patients given aspirin at discharge	100%	100%	100%
Effective Heart Attack Care	Heart attack patients given a prescription for a statin at discharge	97%	98%	98%
Effective Heart Failure Care	Heart failure patients given discharge instructions	92%	98%	94%
Effective Heart Failure Care	Heart failure patients given am evaluation of left ventricular systolic (LVS) function	97%	97%	98%
Effective Heart Failure Care	Heart failure patients given ACE inhibitor or ARB for left ventricular systolic dysfunction (LVSD)	97%	98%	98%
Effective Pneumonia Care	Pneumonia patients whose initial emergency room blood culture was performed prior to the administration of the hospital dose of antibiotics	97%	98%	97%
Effective Pneumonia Care	Pneumonia patients given the most appropriate initial antibiotics	96%	97%	96%
Timely Surgical Care	Outpatients having surgery who got an antibiotic at the right time—within one hour before surgery	98%	99%	99%
Timely Surgical Care	Surgery patients who were given an antibiotic at the right time (within one hour before surgery) to help prevent infection	98%	99%	99%
Timely Surgical Care	Surgery patients whose preventive antibiotics were stopped at the right time (within 24 hours after surgery)	97%	96%	96%

TABLE A.6

CMS Core Measures for Hospitals in Capital City: 2014 Capital City General (CCG) and Osteopathic Medical Center (OMC) (continued)

(continued)

Category	CMS Core Measure	State Benchmark	2014 CCG	2014 OMC
Timely Surgical Care	Patients who got treatment at the right time (within 24 hours before or after their surgery) to help prevent blood clot after certain types of surgery.	97%	98%	98%
Effective Surgical Care	Outpatients having surgery who got the right kind of antibiotic	98%	99%	100%
Effective Surgical Care	Surgery patients who were taking beta blockers before coming to the hospital, who were kept on the beta blockers during the period just before and after the surgery.	96%	96%	96%
Effective Surgical Care	Surgery patients who were given the right kind of antibiotic to help prevent infection	98%	100%	99%
Effective Surgical Care	Heart surgery patients whose blood sugar is kept under good control in the days right after surgery	95%	95%	95%
Effective Surgical Care	Surgery patients whose urinary catheters were removed on the first or second day after surgery	94%	94%	94%
Effective Surgical Care	Patients having surgery who were actively warmed in the operating room or whose body temperature was near normal by the end of surgery	100%	100%	100%
Effective Surgical Care	Surgery patients whose doctor ordered treatments to prevent blood clots after certain types of surgeries	98%	99%	98%
Emergency Department (ED) Care	Average (median) time patient spent in the ED before they were admitted to the hospital as an inpatient (minutes)	Being developed	256	223

(continued)

Category	CMS Core Measure	State Benchmark	2014 CCG	2014 OMC
Emergency Department (ED) Care	Average (median) time patient spent in the ED, after the doctor decided to admit him as an inpatient before leaving the ED for inpatient care (minutes)	Being developed	65	86
Emergency Department (ED) Care	Average time patients spent in the ED before being sent home (minutes)	Being developed	135	156
Emergency Department (ED) Care	Average time patients who came to the ED with broken bones had to wait before receiving pain medication (minutes)	Being developed	35	60
Emergency Department (ED) Care	Percentage of patients who left the ED before being seen	Being developed	6%	8%
Emergency Department (ED) Care	Percentage of patients who came to the ED with stoke symptoms who received brain scans results within 45 minutes of arrival	Being developed	35%	50%
Preventive Care	Patients assessed and given influenza vaccination	95%	99%	97
Preventive Care	Patients assessed and given pneumonia vaccination	93%	93%	93%
Readmission, Complications and Death	Rate of readmission for heart attack		No different	No different
Readmission, Complications and Death	Death rate for heart attack patients		No different	Better
Readmission, Complications and Death	Rate of readmission for heart failure patients		Better	No different

TABLE A.6

CMS Core Measures for Hospitals in Capital City: 2014 Capital City General (CCG) and Osteopathic Medical Center (OMC) (continued)

(continued)

TABLE A.6

CMS Core
Measures for
Hospitals in Capital
City: 2014 Capital
City General (CCG)
and Osteopathic
Medical Center
(OMC)
(continued)

Category	CMS Core Measure	State Benchmark	2014 CCG	2014 OMC
Readmission, Complications and Death	Rate of readmission for pneumonia patients		No different	No different
Readmission, Complications and Death	Death rate for pneumonia patients		No different	No different
Serious Complications and Deaths	Serious complications—rate		Better	No different
Hospital Acquired Conditions	Hospital-acquired conditions		Better	No different
Healthcare Associated Infections	Central line-associated bloodstream infections		No different	No different
Use of Medical Imaging	Outpatients with low back pain who had an MRI without trying recommended treatments first, such as PT	32.9%	36%	37%
Use of Medical Imaging	Outpatients who had a follow-up mammogram or ultrasound within 45 days after a screening mammogram	12.4%	12%	14%
Use of Medical Imaging	Outpatient CT scans of the chest that were "combination" scans	0.3%	0.3%	0.3%
Use of Medical Imaging	Outpatient CT scans of the abdomen that were "combination" scans	0.7%	0.9%	0.1%
Use of Medical Imaging	Outpatients who got cardiac imaging stress tests before low-risk outpatient surgery	Being developed	11%	7%
Use of Medical Imaging	Outpatients with brain CT scans who got a sinus CT scan at the same time	Being developed	4%	4%

(continued)

Category	CMS Core Measure	State Benchmark	2014 CCG	2014 OMC
Patient Survey Results	Patients who reported that their nurses "always" communicated well	84%	92%	88%
Patient Survey Results	Patients who reported that their doctor "always" communicated well	80%	73%	83%
Patient Survey Results	Patients who reported they "always" received help as soon as they wanted	62%	66%	65%
Patient Survey Results	Patients who reported that their pain was "always" well controlled	75%	70%	72%
Patient Survey Results	Patients who reported that staff "always" explained about medicines before giving it to them	69%	79%	74%
Patient Survey Results	Patients who reported that their room and bathroom was "always" clean	73%	72%	74%
Patient Survey Results	Patients who reported that the area around their room was "always" quiet at night	73%	70%	71%
Patient Survey Results	Patients at each hospital who reported "yes," they were given information about what to do during their recovery at home	85%	94%	90%
Patient Survey Results	Patients who gave their hospital a rating of 9 or 10 on a scale from 0 to 10	68%	60%	60%
Patient Survey Results	Patients who reported "yes," they would definitely recommend the hospital	76%	75%	73%

TABLE A.6
CMS Core Measures for Hospitals in Capital City: 2014 Capital City General (CCG) and Osteopathic Medical Center (OMC) (continued)

NOTES: "n/a" means not applicable and the data are either not available or that the number of cases is too small for a legitimate conclusion. "Being developed" means that the core measure remains under development and no standard or benchmark has yet been published. "State" means the statewide mean score. "Better" means better than national average. "No difference" means no statistical difference between the hospital and national averages.

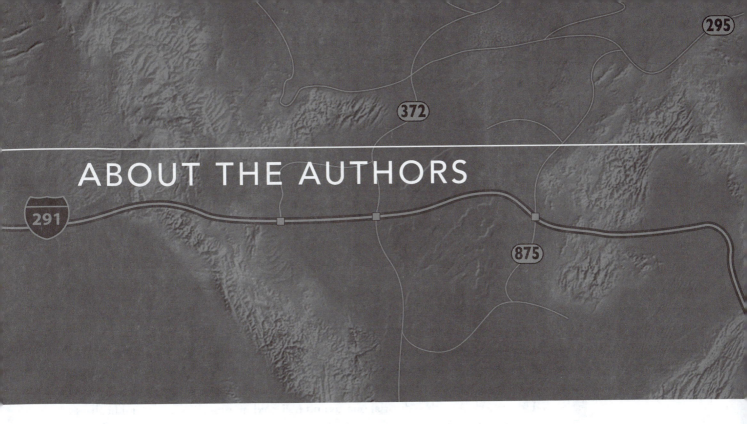

ABOUT THE AUTHORS

Lee F. Seidel, PhD, is professor of health management and policy at the University of New Hampshire (UNH) and visiting professor in the executive MBA in health administration program at the University of Colorado, Denver. He teaches capstone courses in both settings and courses in financial management and healthcare systems at UNH. At UNH he is the founding director of the UNH Center for Teaching and Learning and managed this center for 15 years. The center is a recipient of a national Theodore M. Hesburgh Award. UNH recently awarded Seidel the Jean Brierley Award, its highest honor for effective teaching. He is also the first Association of University Programs in Health Administration (AUPHA) board chair from a baccalaureate program.

Seidel has authored four books and numerous articles on health administration, health administration education, and effective college teaching. His work has been supported by numerous sources, including the WK Kellogg Foundation and the Fund for Improvement of Postsecondary Education of the US Department of Education. Prior to his academic career, he worked with Arthur Andersen and Company and for the Office of the Mayor, City of New York. Seidel holds an MPA and PhD in community systems planning and development with emphasis in health administration from the Pennsylvania State University.

James B. Lewis, ScD, is associate professor of health management and policy at the University of New Hampshire (UNH). At UNH he has taught courses at the baccalaureate and graduate levels in health finance, health marketing, social marketing, strategic planning, strategic management, health reimbursement, managed care, and introduction to the healthcare system. He has also directed the university's undergraduate and graduate programs in health management and public health and served as department chair for several years.

Lewis holds an MBA from Northwestern University and an ScD from the Johns Hopkins School of Hygiene and Public Health. Prior to his academic appointment, he was a healthcare management consultant specializing in strategy and strategic planning, having been a principal with the firm of William M. Mercer and the national manager of healthcare strategic planning for Coopers & Lybrand. In these positions, Lewis provided advice to dozens of healthcare organizations, insurance companies, and purchasers of healthcare services.

Lewis has coauthored three books and approximately 20 journal articles and case studies. He has served on the editorial boards and reviewed manuscripts for several health-related journals. He is a member of the AUPHA and has been a program reviewer at both the undergraduate and graduate level.